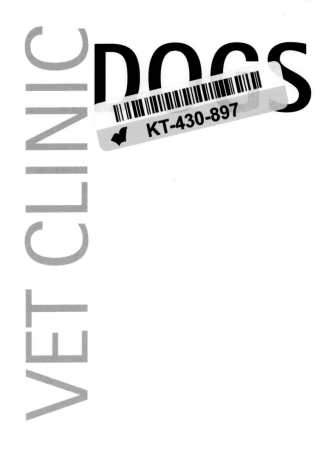

VET CLINIC DOGS

DEDICATION

*I unreservedly
dedicate this book to my wife, Jane,
and our son, Thomas, for their
ceaseless help and support in all
that I do.*

Commissioning Editor: Julian Brown
Project Editor: Tarda Davison-Aitkins
Creative Director: Keith Martin
Executive Art Director: Mark Winwood
Designer: Les Needham
Production Controller: Lee Sargent

First published in Great Britain in 2000
by Hamlyn, a division of
Octopus Publishing Group Limited
2–4 Heron Quays, London E14 4JP

First published in paperback in 2002

ISBN 0 600 60677 5

A catalogue record for this book is available from
the British Library

Printed in China

10 9 8 7 6 5 4 3 2 1

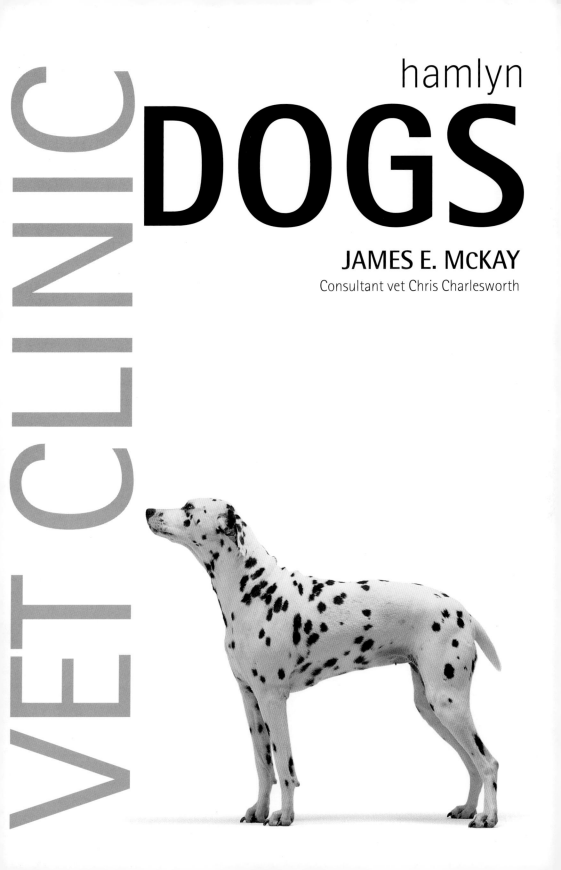

hamlyn
DOGS

JAMES E. MCKAY

Consultant vet Chris Charlesworth

VET CLINIC

Comprehensive
Health Care for DOGS

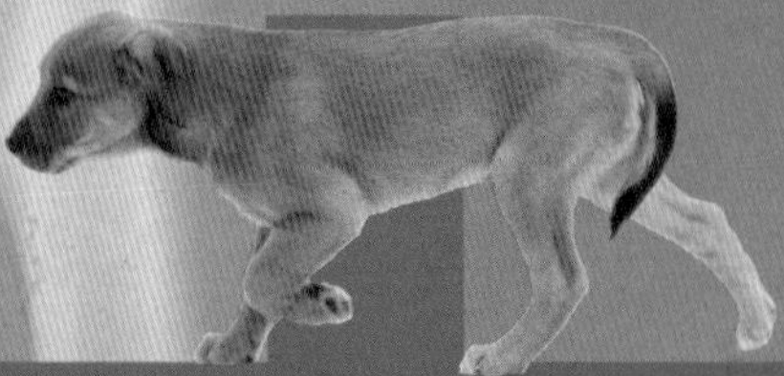

contents

Introduction 6

CHAPTER 1 **Ear conditions**
Aural haematoma 8
Deafness 10
Otitis 12
Ear flap wounds 14
Ear mites 15

CHAPTER 2 **Eye conditions**
Conjunctivitis 17
Abnormal tear production 18
Corneal ulceration 19
Glaucoma 20
Cataract 20
Blindness 21

CHAPTER 3 **Eating and drinking**
Bad breath or halitosis 23
Worn and broken teeth and
    abscesses 24
Retained teeth 26
Difficulty swallowing 26

Diabetes mellitus 28
Vomiting 30
Flatulence 31
Diarrhoea 32
Cystitis 33
Enteritis 34
Constipation 35
Renal failure 36
Urinary incontinence 37
Anal sac disease 38

CHAPTER 4 **Movement**
Lameness 40
Arthritis 42
Spondylosis 42
Paralysis 43
Degenerative disc disease 44
Fractures 46
Dislocation 48
Poor exercise tolerance 49
Vertebral instability 50
Hip dysplasia 50

CHAPTER 5 **Breathing and circulation**
Contagious respiratory disease 53
Chronic bronchial disease 54
Rhinitis 55
Collapsed trachea 56
Pneumonia 57
The circulatory system 58
Heart problems 59
Mitral insufficiency 60
Cardiomyopathy 61
Other heart problems 62
Anaemia 63

CHAPTER 6 **The skin**
Alopecia 65
Fleas 66
Mites 67
Ticks 68
Food allergies 70
Ringworm 71
Pyoderma 72
Seborrhoea 73

CHAPTER 7 **Male dog problems**
Aggression 75
Sexual behaviour 76
Anorchia and cryptorchidism 76
Testicular tumour 77
Anal adenoma 78
Prostate problems 78

CHAPTER 8 **Bitch problems**
The bitch's reproductive system 80
Pseudo pregnancy 81
Pyometra 82
Mammary cancer 83

Mastitis 84
Eclampsia 85
Nymphomania 86
Metritis 86
Vaginal prolapse or hyperplasia 87
Vaginitis 88
Misalliance 88
Toxocara canis 89

CHAPTER 9 **Problems suffered by
   elderly dogs**
Senility 91
Coat problems 92
Incontinence 93
Liver failure 94
Tooth decay 94
Obesity 95

CHAPTER 10 **Other medical disorders**
Behaviour problems 96
Physiological problems 97
Cancer 98
Cushing's disease 99
Epilepsy 100
Euthanasia 101

CHAPTER 11 **Accidents and emergencies**
Quick reference 103
Emergency techniques 104
Serious injuries 106
Major injuries and dangerous
   conditions 110
Minor injuries 117
The first aid kit 120

INDEX 124
ACKNOWLEDGEMENTS 128

Introduction

This book is intended to help you to look after your dog. It explains the symptoms, causes and treatments of many of the more common medical problems that a dog owner is likely to see. The book is divided into sections such as 'Ear conditions', 'Eye conditions' and 'Breathing and circulation' to make it easier for you to look up specific problems. Further information to help the reader is given in the form of an urgency indicator to tell you how important it is to seek veterinary treatment for that particular condition or disease, and tips on any action you as an owner can take to help your dog. There is also a chapter on 'Accident and Emergency' to help you should you need to give first aid to a dog in an emergency situation.

Many medical problems are caused by the attitude of owners to their dogs, and I have also given advice on how to avoid these, by correct feeding, good exercise and awareness of early symptoms of illnesses. Common sense is essential in all animal husbandry, and regular visits to the vet for a check-up on your dog is recommended. You should ensure that your dog is regularly wormed and vaccinated against the commonly occurring diseases in your area. Neutering, too, is worth considering if you do not intend to breed from your dog, as many diseases are only seen in 'entire' dogs and bitches.

Your vet will welcome your questions concerning the health and wellbeing of your dog, and will be happy to explain medical conditions – their causes, treatment and prevention – to you. Vets understand the importance of educating the dog owner, as this leads to dogs being better treated and healthier.

One of the most important ways to keep your dog healthy is to feed him a balanced, good quality diet. It will help maintain him in good condition, and he will be able to fight off infections and disease more easily. The main components of a balanced diet are proteins, vitamins, minerals, carbohydrates, fats and fibre. A dog fed on a truly balanced diet will lead a long, active and healthy life. With the easy availability of a whole range of complete diets for all life stages and lifestyles of dogs, this is easy to achieve.

It is very important that your dog is not overweight, as obesity is linked to many problems and disorders, and an obese dog is far more likely to suffer from certain diseases. Your vet can advise you if you are concerned about your dog's weight.

Most of the treatments given in this book relate to 'normal' veterinary techniques. These are techniques taught to all vets during their training, and have served vets, and the pets for which they care, well over the years. Today, some vets are exploring other techniques and methods of treating animals. Some are now turning to what is termed a holistic approach, where the whole animal is considered, rather than simply the condition(s) that the animal is exhibiting.

One of the approaches which vets are increasingly taking to improve the health of animals is homeopathy. This is a very complicated science, in which the vet administers extremely tiny amounts of substances that are known, in excess, to cause the problem from which the dog is suffering. The mechanism by which homeopathy works is not very well understood, but more and more people are turning to it as an alternative form of treatment. The fact that it does work, often with astonishing effect, ensures that more interest will be taken in this area of veterinary medicine in the future.

Where relevant, this book lists some homeopathic treatments that may help a dog suffering from a particular disorder. If you are interested in having your pet treated by homeopathic techniques, talk it over with your vet, or if your vet appears to be cynical about the subject, contact another vet who has a genuine interest in homeopathy.

This book is not a substitute for taking a sick dog for veterinary treatment. If your dog shows any signs of illness, it is highly advisable that you seek veterinary advice as soon as possible. Delay in some cases can mean the difference between your dog making a speedy and full recovery, or suffering a long and painful disease and, in some cases, death.

If you are ever in doubt about your dog's health, consult your vet immediately.

Please note that throughout this book I have referred to the dog as 'he' but the text applies equally to both the chapters on bitch problems and male dog problems.

I would like to express my thanks and gratitude to Chris Charlesworth, MRCVS, and all of his staff – vets, nurses, and support workers – and his clients and patients for their help in the production of this book.

James McKay

Ear conditions

The ear is made up of three parts, any of which can, and sometimes do, cause problems in a dog.

● **The pinna (plural pinnae)**. This is the outer part of the ear (the flap) which collects and funnels sounds to the ear drum, a white sheet of tissue stretched across the ear canal. The ear drum changes these sounds to vibrations.

● **The middle ear.** This part of the ear contains the ossicles (ear bones), and these transmit the vibrations from the ear drum to the inner ear.

● **The inner ear**. This is where the vibrations are translated into electrical signals, and these signals are then transmitted to the brain, which interprets them as sounds.

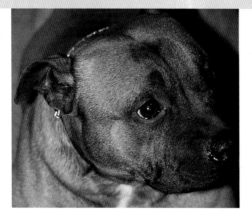

Although breeds of dog with large ears are more susceptible to aural haematoma, any breed can suffer from them.

Aural haematoma

A blood blister on the ear flap.

Symptoms
A lump under the skin of the pinna. This may or may not be painful to the dog.

Underlying causes
When a dog scratches his ears and shakes his head in response to irritation, perhaps caused by fleas or mites, or an ear infection, he may scratch too hard, bang the ear flap against a solid object or simply shake it too vigorously, causing a blood blister. This is the accumulation of fluid between the layers of skin in the ear flap, around the cartilage sheet. There is some evidence

to suggest that in some cases aural haematoma may be caused by the dog's immune system reacting to an infection.

Breeds of dog with large ears – spaniels, golden retrievers and setters – are more susceptible to haematomas than dogs with small ears, but any breed of dog can suffer from them.

DIAGNOSING AURAL HAEMATOMA

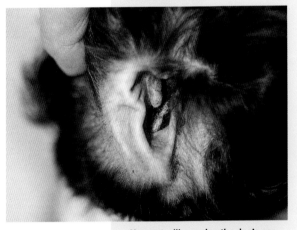

Your vet will examine the dog's ear, both externally, and internally using an otoscope. The otoscope is an instrument fitted with cone-shaped ends of differing sizes, enabling the device to fit snugly into the dog's ear canal. It is used to see inside the ear, and has a magnifying lens and its own light source. The vet can examine the lining of the ear canal, or the ear drum.

Your vet is also likely to examine the rest of the dog, to discover what has made the dog scratch himself so vigorously. The irritants may be fleas or other parasites, or an ear infection.

URGENCY INDICATOR

Aural haematoma is not life-threatening but it is painful for the affected dog, and curing it can be far from simple, so treatment should be started as soon as possible. The condition worsens over time, as the haematoma increases in size and becomes more difficult to treat.

Owner action

Although this condition is not classed as an emergency, your vet should be consulted as soon as possible.

Treatment

It may take your vet more than one attempt to cure the aural haematoma, and different treatments may be tried. These might include inserting a drainage tube into the haematoma, and leaving it in place for several weeks; drawing the fluid out with a syringe (aspiration); or even operating on the dog, using a general anaesthetic and cutting open the ear to flush out the contents of the haematoma.

Antibiotics and/or painkillers are also usually prescribed, and the dog may have to wear an Elizabethan collar.

HOMEOPATHIC TREATMENT: Arnica will help reduce blood loss and tissue damage. Hamamelis will help relieve pain.

COST
This condition can be difficult to treat, and many different treatments may have to be tried before the condition clears up completely, so costs may be quite high.

Deafness

Partial or complete loss of hearing.

Symptoms

The dog may fail to respond to verbal commands, or appear to sleep very soundly, not waking when you call him.

Underlying causes

There are many different causes of deafness in a dog. Deafness is not itself a disease, but a symptom of a problem or disease. In some breeds, such as Dalmatians, cocker spaniels, German shepherd dogs and Old English sheepdogs, deafness is a known and almost expected problem, but it can occur in any breed.

The problem could occur anywhere along the route taken by sounds before they arrive at the brain. This could include a physical blockage of the ear canal, by either a physical agent, swelling(s) or even small tumours, known as polyps. The ear drum itself may be damaged, as may the ossicles.

One of the breeds that suffer from deafness is the German shepherd dog, although the affliction can affect any breed.

DIAGNOSING DEAFNESS

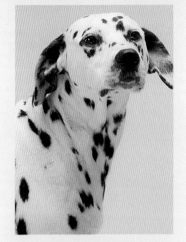

Your vet will examine the dog's ears for obvious physical problems and, if these are not found, he will carry out more tests, sometimes including electronic hearing tests.

Treatment

If there is a blockage, the vet will remove this, and, if possible, treat any underlying problems that may originally have caused the blockage.

If your dog is profoundly and permanently deaf, you will have to face the dilemma that keeping a deaf dog produces. Many people feel that it is possible for the dog to live a fairly normal life, and he may be trained to obey hand signals. However, even if the dog learns to obey hand signals, it will be difficult to get him to look towards you, especially when he has become distracted by something. Some believe that the kindest course of action is for a permanently, profoundly deaf dog to be humanely destroyed. Your own vet will be able to offer advice and guidance on individual cases.

There may be a build-up of fluid in the middle ear, or the problem may be associated with old age. Some animals are born with deformities and abnormalities of the ear.

URGENCY INDICATOR

Not life-threatening, but it is far better to get veterinary advice sooner rather than later.

Owner action

It can often be surprisingly difficult to notice that your dog actually has a hearing problem, since many compensate for their hearing loss, for example by looking more intently at their owners. If you suspect that there may be a problem, try speaking to your dog when he has his back turned, or when his attention is on something he has seen. Also try different types, volumes and pitches of sound.

If you feel that your dog fails these tests, or that they are inconclusive, seek veterinary help.

COST

This will depend on the cause of the deafness, as well as the number of tests needed to diagnose the underlying problem.

Otitis

Inflammation of the skin lining the ear. Otitis is one of the most common conditions seen by vets in dogs, and may occur in one or both ears.

Symptoms
May include a discharge or smell from the ear, regular ear-scratching and head-shaking, and reddening of the inner ear flap and/or the ear hole. The dog may snap at anyone who touches him around the ear.

Underlying causes
Normally, the amount of wax produced in a dog's ear is exactly the same as the amount that is lost naturally. Much of the wax is lost through evaporation of the water from the wax. Problems occur when the ears do not get proper ventilation, as in dogs with large folded ears, such as spaniels, golden retrievers, setters, etc. The flaps prevent adequate water loss, and so the wax builds up. This excess wax causes irritation, and the ear is stimulated to produce even more wax. This leads to ideal conditions for normally harmless fungi and bacteria to grow and prosper, leading in turn to irritation of the skin in the ear. Another major cause of otitis is when the dog has particularly hairy inner ears.

Ear mites (see p. 15), foreign bodies lodged in the ear and skin problems can also cause otitis.

Owner action
Any dog showing any of the symptoms of irritated ears should be taken as soon as possible for examination by a vet: immediately if you suspect that your dog may have a foreign body lodged in his ear. *Never* attempt to remove any such blockage yourself, as you may damage the dog's ear permanently. Do not put any liquid, ointment

If the vet is unable to use his otoscope properly he may apply ear drops to the inside of the ear. Gentle massaging of the ear will allow the drops to do their work.

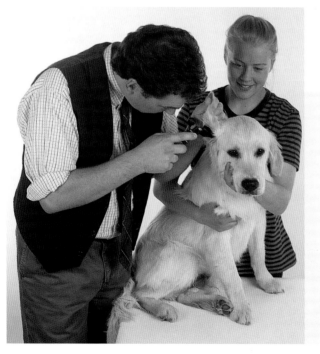

DIAGNOSING OTITIS

Because of the build-up of wax, it may not be possible for your vet to use an otoscope properly. If ear mites have caused the irritation, these may not be seen by the otoscope, as they dislike light and hide under bits of wax when the light is shone in the ear.

Your vet may take a sample of the discharge and/or wax from the ear, and send these for laboratory examination. This will help pinpoint both the problem and the correct and most efficient treatment.

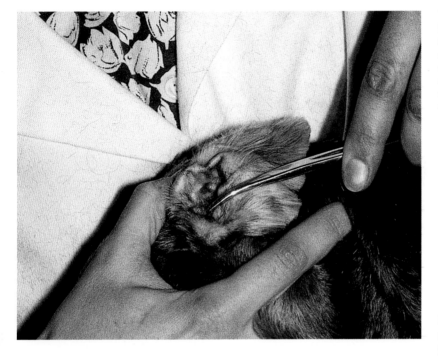

The plucking of the hairs inside a dog's ears must only be carried out by an experienced person, otherwise damage may be done to the dog's ears.

URGENCY INDICATOR

Even though otitis is not a serious condition, if it is not properly treated it can become chronic, causing severe problems, and damage to parts of the dog's ear.

or other medication inside the dog's ears without the express direction of your vet, and do not attempt to insert any solid object into the dog's ear, including cotton buds, which may also damage the dog's ear. Even the discharge from the dog's ear should not be interfered with until your vet has had a chance to see it, as examination of this may give the vet some clues as to the origins of the ear problem.

Treatment

Treatment may include having the dog's ear syringed (washed out), or the application of a topical medicine (one put directly into the ear), such as ear drops or ointment. Very often more than one of these medicines will be needed: one for, say, ear mites, and another (an anti-inflammatory) for the irritation that the mites are causing. Whatever medications are prescribed, it is important that you administer them exactly as you are instructed, and finish the complete course of treatment.

In serious cases of recurring otitis, the vet may have to operate on the dog to improve the ear ventilation. If the dog has particularly hairy inner ears, the vet may recommend that the ears are plucked on a regular basis. Prevention of the condition is far better than cure.

⊘ HOMEOPATHIC TREATMENT: Psorinum, sulphur or conium given internally will make the ear hostile to mites.

◔ COST

Unlikely to be high if caught in the early stages.

Ear flap wounds

Scratches or tears to the ear flaps.

Symptoms

It is highly likely that any ear wound, no matter how minor, will bleed a great deal. Even if the actual wound does not cause the dog any real pain, the irritation of blood running down the ear is likely to cause him to scratch at his ear and shake his head.

Underlying causes

Ear flaps are often bitten and scratched when dogs fight. While it is unlikely that your dog's ears will become damaged by plants such as brambles, it is quite common for dogs (particularly those with long ears, such as spaniels) to damage their ears on barbed wire or when scavenging in old tin cans etc.

Owner action

Always muzzle the dog before starting treatment, and put on a collar and lead. With someone restraining the dog, the wounds should be cleaned, using saline solution made by dissolving one tablespoon of table salt in 0.5 litre (18 fl oz) of warm water. Once cleaned, it will be possible to see the extent of the damage to the ear flap. If this is significant, then veterinary treatment should be sought, as the wounds may need suturing (stitching).

COST

Minor ear injuries, treated adequately soon after they occur, will cost little to treat.

URGENCY INDICATOR

If these wounds are not treated adequately, they may become infected and far more serious.

Treatment

Once the wounds have been cleaned with saline solution, if they are minor they should be covered with antiseptic ointment, cream or powder. If the wounds look inflamed within a few days of the injury, consult the vet, as the dog may need treatment with antibiotics.

To keep the ear flap in place, cut one leg from a pair of tights and, once some padding has been placed around the affected ear flap, place the leg of the tights over the dog's head, in such a way that the ear is held flat to the dog's head. Failing this, a carefully wound bandage can be used to hold the ear flap flat against the dog's head.

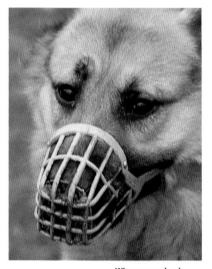

Whenever a dog is injured and in pain, there is a risk that he may bite you. Apply a muzzle to the dog before you begin to treat him.

Ear mites

Insect parasites common in dogs.

Symptoms
Persistent ear-scratching and head-shaking.

Underlying causes
Ear mites, *Otodectes cynotis*, which are common in dogs and also in wild rodents.

Owner action
Seek veterinary advice in all cases of ear mites, loss of balance etc. Do not try to treat the condition yourself. It is important that all animals that have been in contact with the infected dog are also treated, as ear mites can infect other animals who may not show any symptoms for some time. The treatment needs to last for at least three weeks, otherwise the eggs laid in the dog's coat will not be killed.

Treatment
In mild cases, ear drops will be prescribed. Anti-inflammatory drugs may also be prescribed if the dog's ears are irritated due to the action of the mites.

DIAGNOSING EAR MITES

A build-up of wax in the ears, dotted with black specks, is an indication that a dog may have ear mites; the black specks are probably spots of dried blood. The ear mites are usually white or colourless and are not visible to the naked eye – a magnifying lens or otoscope is required, although otoscopes may not be able to detect them as the mites hide under pieces of wax.

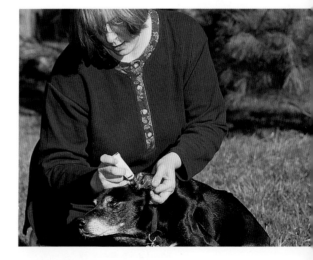

HOMEOPATHIC TREATMENT:
Psorinum or sulphur will help relieve irritation, but normal veterinary treatments must be used to get rid of the mites.

Ear drops, prescribed by a vet for the specific dog ailment, are usually all that is needed to treat an ear mite infection.

URGENCY INDICATOR

If left untreated, the irritation caused by mites will cause the dog to scratch, sometimes until his ears actually bleed. The mites can move down the ear canal and infect the middle ear; such an infection will cause the affected animal to lose his sense of balance. The dog may simply be unable to hold his head straight or, in more serious cases, may constantly fall over.

RELATED CONDITIONS WHICH MAY PRODUCE SIMILAR SIGNS

Many similar conditions can give the general symptoms of an ear-mite infestation, so it is essential that your vet diagnoses the problem and treats it accordingly.

COST
Mites are easily treated if caught early enough, and so the cost will be quite low.

Eye conditions

The eyeball or globe consists of three layers:

- **the outer layer, which includes the cornea;**
- **the middle layer, which contains the iris; and**
- **the inner layer, the retina.**

The transparent part of the eyeball, which allows your dog to see out, is known as the cornea. Through this, you can see the iris and the pupil. The middle layer contains the ligament which holds the lens. This lens focuses light on the retina, which contains light-sensitive cells, called rods and cones. Cones are responsible for colour vision. Within the retina lies the optic nerve, through which the eye sends signals to the brain.

The eye is a very complex and vital organ. Any injury or damage to or abnormality of the eye should be referred to a vet immediately. Failure to act quickly may result in the dog suffering permanent damage to the eye or even total blindness.

Some eye conditions are hereditary, and some breeds are more prone to certain eye problems than others. If you are purchasing a pedigree dog, then you should check with the breeders to ensure that the puppy's parents have both been screened for any hereditary eye problems. However, even mongrel dogs can suffer from eye problems.

WARNING: NEVER TRY TO TREAT ANY EYE PROBLEMS YOURSELF: ALWAYS SEEK VETERINARY ADVICE.

Conjunctivitis

Inflammation of the membrane on the inner eyelids and over the eyeball, or the third eyelid (the nictitating membrane). This is the major cause of reddened eyes, and may affect one or both eyes. It may be acute (appears rapidly) or chronic (appears slowly, lasts a long time and is resistant to treatment). Even relatively mild cases of conjunctivitis can lead to the affected dog injuring his eye when scratching at the irritation. In many cases of conjunctivitis, there are underlying conditions that can be very dangerous for the affected dog.

Symptoms

Include reddened eyes, increased blinking, a thick discharge from the corner of one or both eyes, 'crying' (increased tear production), half-closed eyes, constant scratching around the eyes, or rubbing of the face on hard objects or along the floor.

Underlying causes

Conjunctivitis can be caused by allergies, infections (bacterial, fungal or viral), physical damage (for example, from thorns, grass seeds or other foreign bodies in the eye), inadequate tear production or ingrowing eyelashes.

Working gundogs, who have to push through thick, dense foliage in their everyday life, are at risk from conjunctivitis caused by a foreign body in the eye, such as a thorn or a grass seed, but any dog can pick up these foreign bodies quite easily. Pekinese dogs and King Charles spaniels, which have large, bulging eyes, are vulnerable to eye damage.

Owner action

Look out for any reddening of the dog's eyes. If you believe that there is a foreign body in the eye, do not attempt to remove it with a solid object such as a finger, cotton bud or tweezers (forceps), because

URGENCY INDICATOR

If the dog shows no signs of improvement from his original symptoms within 24 hours, or the eyes have reddened and become weepy, take him to the vet as soon as possible.

HOMEOPATHIC TREATMENT:
The treatment of this condition is well established, and enjoys a high degree of success. A great number of remedies can be used on conjunctivitis, including euphrasia, aconite, pulsatilla and Sanicula.

COST
Not high in mild cases. If left, the condition will worsen, and the cost of treatment will increase.

DIAGNOSING CONJUNCTIVITIS

The vet will remove any discharge from around the eye and then carefully examine the dog's eye(s) using an ophthalmoscope. This has a built-in light with several filters and lenses which can be used to examine both the internal and external eye. The eyeball surface will be examined in more detail. Samples may be taken from the dog's eye(s) for laboratory analysis, to help discover the cause of the problem.

you may cause far more damage to the eye. Pour about a litre (1¾ pints) of warm water very gently over the affected eye(s). Using a piece of cotton wool soaked in warm water, wipe around but not on the eye, removing any debris or discharge.

Treatment

Depending on the cause of the problem, the vet may prescribe antibiotics in the form of eye ointments or drops, and/or anti-inflammatory drugs, either topical (applied directly into the eye) or by mouth. It is important that any such treatment is given regularly, as directed, and that the course is completed, or the problem may prove extremely difficult to clear up, and may recur regularly.

RELATED CONDITIONS WHICH MAY PRODUCE SIMILAR SYMPTOMS

Reddening of the eye can be caused by several other conditions, and also by a foreign object in the dog's eye. It is therefore important that you have your dog examined by a vet before attempting any treatments.

Abnormal tear production

Overflowing of tears onto the dog's face, known as epiphora. Tears are one of nature's ways of flushing dirt and debris from the eyes, working together with the eyelids, and so play an important role in keeping the eyes healthy.

Symptoms

Tears normally drain away through the tear duct, a tube-like vessel which connects the eye with the nose. When this flow is impeded, the tears overflow onto the dog's face. It is most obvious on dogs with white faces. Toy breeds are extremely susceptible to the problem, and dogs with large, droopy eyelids also tend to suffer from epiphora more than the average dog.

Underlying causes

The usual cause of epiphora is one or both tear ducts being blocked. This blockage could be due to a foreign body becoming lodged in the tear duct, an infection, facial injury, scarring following an injury, or excessive mucous production. The tear ducts may be unable to function correctly due to a congenital defect (one present from birth). Irritation of the eye may also cause abnormal tear production.

Owner action

Any dog showing signs of tear-staining or a long-term weepy eye should be examined by a vet.

Treatment

Where the cause of the problem is an infection, antibiotics will be prescribed – ointment, drops or medicine by mouth. Where the problem is caused by a lack of drainage, the vet may decide to anaesthetize or heavily sedate the dog, and wash out the blocked tear duct using a canula, a very fine tube that is attached to a syringe.

Prevention is better than cure, and a dog's eyes should be washed regularly with warm water to remove debris from the area before it can become a problem. This is particularly important if the dog is one of the breeds or types that is more susceptible to these problems.

HOMEOPATHIC TREATMENT: Euphrasia is one of the most useful treatments for this condition.

DIAGNOSING ABNORMAL TEAR PRODUCTION

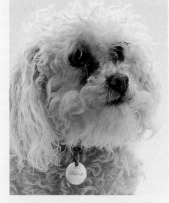

One of the procedures employed by vets to observe the amount of drainage from an eye is to put fluoroscein (a dye) into the affected eye(s). If the tear ducts are draining the eyes as they should be, the dye will come down the dog's nostrils.

COST

A common condition that should not need expensive treatment, if treated early.

Corneal ulceration

An ulcer on the cornea, formed when the surface, which is usually very smooth, becomes damaged.

Symptoms
Include increased blinking, increased tear production, reddened eye, dislike of bright lights, discomfort or pain, a change of colour in the cornea (to an opaque blue-grey) and swollen conjunctiva (the membrane that covers the front of the eye).

Underlying causes
The damage to the cornea may be in the form of a scratch, damage from a blocked tear duct reducing the production of tears, a foreign body in the eye, an infection, a tumour, or damage caused by ingrowing eyelids. One type of ulcer is caused by *Pseudomonas* bacteria, and these are capable of spreading at such a fast rate, and are so aggressive, that they are known as 'melting ulcers'.

Although any dog can suffer from corneal ulcers, they are more likely to occur in those breeds with bulging eyes (for example, King Charles spaniels), and also older dogs. The ulcers are very painful and can soon spread, so must be treated by a vet as soon as possible. Some ulcers can rupture the cornea, causing extremely serious damage.

Owner action
It is best not to attempt any treatment of your dog's eyes; leave this to the vet, as serious and often irreparable damage can be done all too easily.

Treatment
Any foreign body found in the eye will be removed by the vet, and antibiotics will be administered for infection. As the prob-

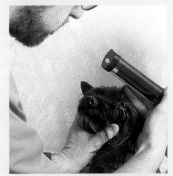

DIAGNOSING CORNEAL ULCERATION

The vet will administer fluoroscein to the eye, which will stick to the ulcer, but run off the unaffected areas of the cornea. Ultraviolet light shone into the eye will make the dye fluoresce and enable the ulcer to be seen.

lem will cause the dog some discomfort, an Elizabethan collar may need to be fitted in order to prevent the eye being rubbed which would cause further damage to it.

In a small minority of cases, where the corneal ulcer will not heal, the affliction may be treated surgically, either by cauterizing the ulcer or surgically removing damaged tissue around it. A flap of healthy conjunctiva may have to be fixed over the ulcer for a few days.

HOMEOPATHIC TREATMENT: Mercurial remedies may be effective.

COST Eye damage can require specialist veterinary treatment, and this could be expensive.

Glaucoma

A build-up of fluid in the eye leading to the pressure of the fluid contents of the eye increasing.

Symptoms
Eventually swelling and bulging of the affected eye(s), and blindness. The dog will be in pain and may shy away from light, as the condition makes the pupils dilate excessively and continuously.

Underlying causes
Glaucoma is usually caused by a disease of the eye, the most common being lens dislocation. This is where the lens in the eye moves forward. This movement may either be the result of trauma, or because of a hereditary weakness. The latter is quite common in Sealyhams and many rough-haired terriers.

Owner action
Never try to treat eye problems at home. Seek veterinary treatment.

Treatment
Depending on the underlying cause and severity of the condition, surgery may be needed. In some cases, drug therapy is effective. The drugs used reduce tear production, dilate the pupil and help to improve the drainage from the eye.

URGENCY INDICATOR

Not life-threatening, but as with all eye problems, it is best to consult a vet early.

HOMEOPATHIC TREATMENT:
Symphytum and helleborus.

COST
If surgery is involved, costs will be higher than for drug therapy.

DIAGNOSING GLAUCOMA

The vet will physically examine the dog's eyes. If your dog is referred to a veterinary eye specialist, this vet may measure the pressure of the fluid in the dog's eyes.

Cataract

An opacity of the lens (or the capsule that surrounds it) that may affect one or both eyes, making it difficult for the dog to see things normally. Most cataracts get gradually worse.

Symptoms
A slight greying of the eyes is quite normal as a dog grows older, but it may also be the first indication that a cataract is developing. Where the cataracts are hereditary or caused by the dam's poor diet, they will start to appear when a puppy is just a few weeks old, and progressively worsen until the dog is totally blind. This is usually at two to three years of age, but may happen to dogs as young as one.

As the condition worsens, the affected dog will have greater difficulty leading a normal life. He may bump into objects, such as furniture and doors, and will be extremely anxious and stressed in unfamiliar surroundings.

URGENCY INDICATOR

Not life-threatening, but with all eye conditions, obtain veterinary advice as soon as possible.

Underlying causes
Many dogs develop cataracts in their old age. Others have hereditary cataracts, while some cataracts develop due to poor nutrition of the dam in pregnancy. Diabetes mellitus (see p. 28) is a common cause of cataracts in dogs. Although highly unlikely, cataracts may be caused by a severe trauma, which disturbs the circulation within the eye. Certain breeds of

DIAGNOSING CATARACTS

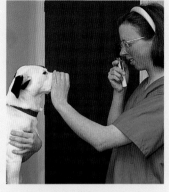

The dog's eyes will be examined using an ophthalmoscope.

dog are more susceptible to hereditary cataracts than others.

Owner action

Any dog suspected of suffering from cataracts must be examined by a vet as soon as possible.

Treatment

Depending on what is found during the eye examination, the dog may be sent for further examination by a veterinary eye specialist. Surgery may be necessary.

HOMEOPATHIC TREATMENT:
To treat the cloudy lens – sulphur. In cases involving injury or an old dog – conium. Where the condition has degenerated following surgery – senega. For long-term treatment – silicea 30.

COST
If surgery is involved, the costs may be quite high.

Blindness

There are degrees of blindness, although the term blind is usually only used when the dog can see nothing at all, or perhaps just light and dark.

Symptoms

Your dog may walk into everyday objects, or may have difficulty finding you, especially if you are in a group of several people. This will probably not affect him finding his food etc., as he will compensate for his poor vision by using his sense of smell even more than usual. It is quite common for an elderly dog to have more problems with his eyesight in bright light and also in darkness, and he may become reluctant to venture out at such times.

Underlying causes

A variety, from injury to hereditary diseases and conditions. As dogs age, it is quite common for a bluish colour to appear in the eyes; this is a normal consequence of ageing, and may lead to the dog's eyesight deteriorating.

Treatment

Totally dependent upon the causes of the sight loss, but many cases of total blindness are not treatable.

DIAGNOSING BLINDNESS

Physical examination of the dog's eyes, with the use of an ophthalmoscope.

URGENCY INDICATOR

Because eyes are so complex, it is vitally important that all eye conditions and injuries are referred to a vet immediately.

Eating and drinking

The dog's digestive system breaks down food from complex foodstuffs to simple compounds, which the body can then absorb and use. Any waste products are excreted.

The digestive system starts at the mouth.

● The teeth are used to hold the food and break, rip or cut up the food into smaller pieces.

● These pieces are then manipulated by the tongue, and mixed with saliva, which moistens and lubricates the food and begins the digestive process.

● Dogs do not chew their food: it is simply cut up by the shearing action of the teeth, and then the smaller lumps are swallowed.

● Like small children, many dogs also use their mouths to investigate the world around them. As a result, they often suffer problems with the mouth and teeth. As teeth are used and abused on a daily basis, they become worn and, in some cases, damaged and broken. Diseases of the teeth and gums are referred to by vets as periodontal diseases.

The swallowed food is pushed down the pharynx (the area at the back of the throat) by muscular contractions, known as peristalsis, until it enters the stomach. In wolves, the wild ancestors of the domestic dog, the stomach was used as a storage vessel, and would have held several days' food. Even domestic dogs still seem to possess this bottomless pit. However, if the stomach is overfilled, the dog will vomit.

In the stomach, the food is mixed with gastric juices, and more of the food is broken down. From the stomach, food passes into the small intestine, where further digestion occurs, and where many of the products of this digestion (amino acids, fatty acids and sugars) are absorbed. From the small intestine, the remnants of the food pass into the large intestine, where water, electrolytes and water-soluble vitamins are absorbed.

Bad breath or halitosis

One of the most common mouth problems suffered by dogs. Most dogs show symptoms before they are three years old.

Symptoms

Bad breath is often a symptom of periodontal disease (disease of the gums and/or teeth). Other signs of periodontal disease can include swollen, tender gums, a loss of appetite and excessive drooling. Plaque and calculus (a build-up of minerals) on a dog's teeth can lead to heart and kidney diseases if left untreated. Yellow-brown stains on the teeth where they meet the gums are a classic symptom.

Underlying causes

Bad breath is often a symptom of periodontal disease. Food sticking on or between the teeth will attract bacteria which will decay the food.

Owner action

Take your dog for regular veterinary check-ups. Frequent cleaning of a dog's teeth can prove beneficial, both as a preventative measure, and also as a way of inspecting the dog's teeth, and finding small problems while they can still be dealt with.

It is advisable to brush your dog's teeth regularly. Use a soft human toothbrush, but *never* use human toothpaste. Brushing the dog's teeth should begin during puppyhood, so the dog becomes used to the treatment. To begin with, simply use a brush dipped into warm water. Holding the mouth closed, place the brush head in the dog's cheek for a few seconds, speaking softly and reassuringly the whole time. Repeat this with the other cheek. Every day, the period should be extended until the dog is no longer concerned about the brush. At this stage,

DIAGNOSING PERIODONTAL DISEASE

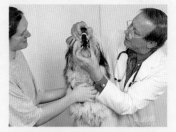

The vet will examine the dog's mouth, looking for obvious problems such as inflammation of the gums or the build-up of calculus or plaque. In some cases, the vet may spray a 'disclosing solution' into the dog's mouth. This solution works in the same way as disclosing solutions for humans, revealing areas of plaque build-up by staining them.

begin to move the brush in a small circle, starting with the back teeth, as these are less sensitive than the front teeth. In a couple of weeks you should be able to brush both the front and back teeth without causing the dog any concern. Then you can introduce small amounts of canine toothpaste. Rubber finger stalls may also be used instead of a toothbrush.

Treatment

If your dog suffers from inflammation of the gums (gingivitis), then it may be helpful to use an antiseptic spray in his mouth. Ask the vet for advice on this.

Your dog's diet will influence the state of his teeth. Feeding mainly soft, tinned food may adversely affect the teeth; it is much better to give at least some crunchy food (kibble or biscuit-type feed) at every mealtime. Large, bare bones provide no benefit and may even damage the teeth and/or gums. A regular supply of chewy 'rawhide' will help keep the dogs teeth and gums in good condition.

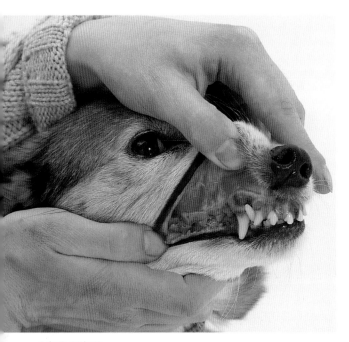

A dog's teeth are essential for his day-to-day living, and so any damage should be investigated and, if necessary, veterinary advice sought.

While not life-threatening, broken teeth are extremely painful, and should be treated as an emergency. Seek veterinary help as soon as possible. Failure to do so may result in further damage and infection. Worn teeth are a natural result of ageing, and are not a real problem, unless they are obviously causing the dog pain or making it difficult for him to eat. If this is the case, seek urgent veterinary advice. If the worn teeth are not causing severe problems to your dog, mention them to your vet at your next routine appointment.

Worn and broken teeth and abscesses

Teeth wear down through natural usage, but may also get broken. Worn teeth, on the whole, present no real problem to the dog, but a broken tooth will cause intense pain, suffering and distress.

DIAGNOSING WORN OR BROKEN TEETH

Two of you will be needed to look inside the dog's mouth. A small torch is essential. Be very careful not to get bitten, as the dog will be in pain, and may resent anyone poking around in its mouth. Your vet may use X-ray examinations to confirm a diagnosis of an abscess.

Symptoms

Broken teeth are obvious when you see them, but they may be at the rear of the mouth, so be on the lookout for any abnormal behaviour which may be linked with pain in the dog's mouth. This may include difficulty eating, leading to a reluctance even to try to eat. In some cases where the dog's tooth is broken, the dog may try to eat, but will yelp as soon as a bite of the food is taken. This calls for a close investigation of the dog's mouth by a vet.

A small, almost unnoticeable swelling on the side of the dog's face may indicate an abscess in the root of one of the teeth, called an apical abscess. The teeth most often affected are the upper carnassials, the dog's largest teeth, situated at the back of the mouth, where human molars are. An abscess on one of these teeth is known as a malar abscess. An abscess will probably not be obvious to the dog's owner, as it is the roots of the tooth that are damaged and not the tooth itself.

Underlying causes

Worn teeth, as well as being the result of ordinary wear and tear, may be due to excessive softness of the teeth, some mal-formation of the jaws, or even the direction in which the teeth are growing. Such problems may have existed since birth.

Broken teeth can be caused by accidents, particularly RTAs (road traffic accidents), and even by a dog chewing on a door (such as his kennel door). Throwing stones for your dog to fetch is another, all too common, cause of broken teeth.

There appear to be two main causes of apical abscesses – damage to the tooth itself, and damage to the blood supply to the root of the tooth. Both types of damage are usually caused by the dog chewing on hard objects, such as large bones, and the dogs involved are usually middle-aged to old, although this problem can afflict a dog of any age and any breed. Whatever the cause, apical abscesses will not cure themselves, and veterinary treatment must be sought.

Owner action

If the dog exhibits symptoms of teeth problems, even if you cannot see any damage, seek veterinary advice, as the problem may be dangerous and painful. Do not attempt to feed your dog until your vet has examined the problem, and then take advice on the type and consistency of food.

Treatment

Broken teeth may be capped to seal them against bits of food or other items working their way into the damaged tooth and to prevent infection, which may cause even more problems and pain. In the case of abscesses, the source of the infection must be removed for the dog to make a complete recovery, and it is normal for the tooth to be removed and the dog placed on a course of antibiotics. It is important that any such treatment is given regularly, as directed, and that the course is completed. Painkillers may also be prescribed for the dog.

In a few cases, dogs suffering from dental problems may be referred to specialist dentistry vets.

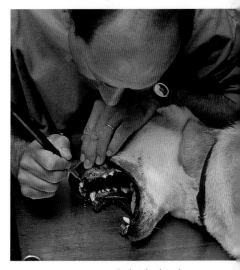

Canine dentistry is invariably carried out with the dog under a general anaesthetic. Your vet may refer you to a specialist.

💲 COST

Severe dental problems and injuries can be quite expensive to treat. Canine dentistry is a specialized discipline, and, as in humans, a costly exercise. All dentistry on dogs needs to be conducted under a general anaesthetic, and this adds to the overall cost of treatment.

RELATED CONDITIONS WHICH MAY PRODUCE SIMILAR SYMPTOMS

Many diseases of the mouth may exhibit symptoms which are very much alike. You should consult your vet if you suspect any such problems. ℹ️

Retained teeth

Milk (deciduous) teeth may not all be shed when the dog starts to get his adult (permanent) teeth. These retained teeth may cause problems for the dog.

Symptoms
May include reddened gums, bloody saliva and abnormal drooling. Where the front or canine teeth are affected, the problem is usually visually obvious, but this may not be the case when the teeth are at the sides or to the rear of the dog's mouth.

Underlying causes
At about 12 weeks of age the dog begins to shed his 28 deciduous teeth, which are gradually replaced by 42 adult teeth. Sometimes, rather than the adult tooth pushing out the milk tooth, the adult tooth may grow in an abnormal direction, often trapping the milk tooth, which is then permanently retained. This may occur with a single tooth, or with several in the dog's mouth, and is often a hereditary problem. It can cause permanent damage to the dog's jaw, and even in less severe cases may still result in pain and distress for the dog.

Owner action
Do not try to treat this condition yourself, but consult your vet as soon as you notice a problem.

Treatment
The retained teeth will need to be removed by surgery. After the operation, the dog may be put on a course of antibiotics and painkillers, and his food may need to be liquidized for a few days.

Difficulty swallowing

This could indicate one of several possible conditions, including pharyngitis or tonsillitis, or even a blockage of the digestive system. Pharyngitis is the inflammation of the pharynx, the area at the back of the dog's throat, while tonsillitis is the inflammation of the tonsils.

Symptoms
These include coughing or retching (as if the throat is blocked), loss of appetite (even though the dog is hungry) and difficulty in swallowing even water.

Underlying causes
Both pharyngitis and tonsillitis can be caused by a viral infection, a bacterial infection following damage to the area done by a foreign body, periodontal (gum)

URGENCY INDICATOR

It is important that any retained milk teeth are removed as soon as possible.

◔ **COST**

As mentioned earlier, canine dental work is a very specialized discipline which can be quite expensive.

DIAGNOSING RETAINED TEETH

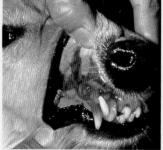

Retained teeth are easily seen in the dog's mouth, and this is one of the potential problems your vet will be looking out for during your dog's annual check-up.

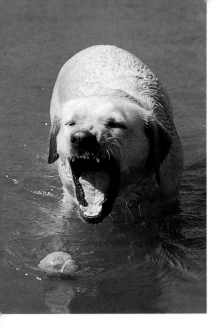

If you notice your dog coughing or retching this could mean he is experiencing swallowing difficulties.

Owner action

Observe your dog, and note his actions. Ensure that he is given sufficient water to drink, to prevent dehydration.

Treatment

A course of antibiotics, which must be given regularly and until the course is completed, will usually clear up any infection of the tonsils or the pharynx.

Even if the vet suspects a blockage of the digestive system, they may not begin treatment immediately, preferring to observe the dog for some time first. Once the diagnosis is confirmed, surgery may be the preferred option.

disease or other factors. Tonsillitis is particularly common in puppies and young dogs, and pharyngitis may occur in any dog of any breed or age.

COST

Depends entirely on the underlying causes and consequent treatment. If surgery is involved, costs may be high.

URGENCY INDICATOR

If you suspect your dog is suffering from any blockage of the digestive system or a problem which is preventing him from swallowing food, it is vital that immediate veterinary investigation is carried out, as a blockage can be life-threatening.

DIAGNOSING TONSILLITIS AND PHARYNGITIS

When inflamed, the dog's tonsils, which are not usually conspicuous, are very obvious, appearing as two very bright red lumps. X-rays will almost always be taken to confirm any diagnosis, before surgery is undertaken. If your dog is suffering from pharyngitis, the lining at the back of the throat will be red and inflamed. Inflammation of the pharynx or tonsils will block the throat.

RELATED CONDITIONS WHICH MAY PRODUCE SIMILAR SYMPTOMS

Periodontal disease can make it painful for the dog to eat or swallow.

A foreign body or other blockage in the digestive system is also a common cause of loss of appetite in a dog. Typically, a dog may chew and swallow stones, paper, wood, bone, small balls, plastic toys and other such objects which become lodged in the digestive system. Such a blockage will cause a variety of symptoms, which include excessive drooling, loss of appetite, regurgitation of food, vomiting, swelling of the abdomen and constipation.

Heart disease is another possible cause of loss of appetite (see p. 59 and 62). In bitches who have had several heats, pyometra may be a reason for loss of appetite (see p. 82), while older dogs may be suffering from liver failure (see p. 94).

Diabetes mellitus

A hormonal condition in which the dog is unable to control his blood sugar levels.

Symptoms

An increase in the dog's appetite, particularly if coupled with other symptoms such as an increase in his thirst, an increase in the amount of urine passed, lethargy, weight loss and maybe cataracts (see p. 20). Very often, symptoms of diabetes mellitus are seen in bitches just after they have started oestrus.

Underlying causes

Diabetes mellitus or 'sugar diabetes' is caused by lack of insulin (produced by the pancreas) or an increase in blood sugar levels (hyperglycaemia). The underlying problem may be quite serious, as it may indicate that the dog's pancreas is not producing enough insulin, perhaps due to an abnormality of the pancreas or through the natural ageing of the organ. In some breeds, including the German shepherd dog, Labrador retrievers, Rottweilers and Samoyeds, the condition is thought to be hereditary. It can, however, occur in almost any dog, most commonly those over eight years of age. Due to the increased levels of progesterone (a hormone) in the blood during phantom or pseudo-pregnancies (see p. 81), unspayed bitches are said to be more then three times more susceptible to diabetes mellitus, and obese dogs of either sex are also at increased risk.

A strict diet may be called for with a dog suffering from diabetes mellitus; it is important that you ensure that your dog adheres strictly to any prescribed diet.

Dogs with diabetes mellitus will need to have samples of their urine tested regularly so the correct treatment can be provided.

DIAGNOSING DIABETES MELLITUS

Blood and urine tests will show the levels of glucose present in the dog's system, while ultrasound and X-ray examinations will show the physical state of the dog's pancreas.

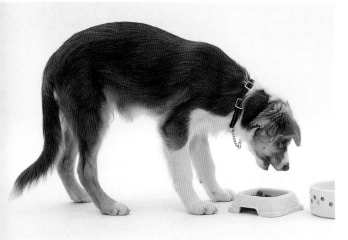

COST

Treatment for this condition is likely to be long term, as your dog may need regular insulin injections and other treatment, so the full costs in time and money will be fairly high.

Your dog's glucose levels will need to be tested every morning. A urine sample will be required in order to calculate the amount of insulin required.

Owner action

Take any dog showing symptoms of diabetes for examination by a vet as soon as possible.

Treatment

Treatment of the condition can be completely successful, provided that the vet is consulted before the condition becomes chronic. It will depend upon the results of all the tests, and the type and cause of the diabetes mellitus. Possible treatments the vet may prescribe include weight loss, spaying, insulin, medication, a special diet and increased exercise. Whatever the treatment, it will inevitably involve you in quite a lot of work over a prolonged period of time. Typically, you will need to collect and test a sample of urine from your dog every morning to check the glucose levels, calculate the amount of insulin needed and administer it by injection, feed your dog an extremely regulated diet at specific times, and ensure he has a proper exercise routine. Your vet will advise you on all of these matters.

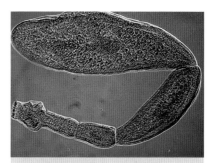

RELATED CONDITIONS WHICH MAY PRODUCE SIMILAR SYMPTOMS

Diabetes insipidus is caused by a lack of anti-diuretic hormone – ADH – (produced in the dog's pituitary glands), or the failure of the kidneys to respond to this hormone. ADH normally helps concentrate the dog's urine when it needs to conserve water. The production of ADH is increased when there is little water intake, and decreased when the dog drinks large quantities of water, thus controlling the body's water balance.

Symptoms of diabetes insipidus include polydipsia (an excessive thirst) and polyuria (production of large amounts of urine). Depending upon which form of diabetes insipidus is present, treatment may involve the administration of ADH to the affected dog; this is introduced into the dog's system via nasal drops.

Many of the conditions associated with diabetes mellitus are also common symptoms of other, less serious, diseases. For example, an increased appetite and/or weight loss may be indications of an infestation of endoparasites, such as tape worms. However, if your dog shows any of the symptoms described earlier, veterinary advice should be sought as soon as possible. ⓘ

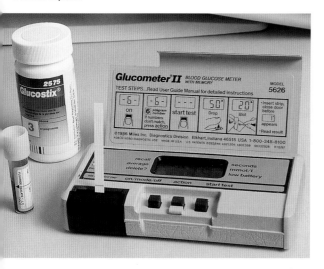

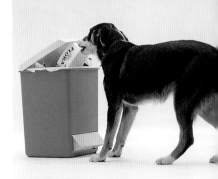

Vomiting

A symptom of another condition, not an illness itself.

Many dogs will scavenge given the opportunity. Ensure that your dog cannot steal rubbish and left-overs from the rubbish bin.

Symptoms

Every reader will recognize the signs of vomiting. Vomiting is a muscular reflex action, resulting in expulsion, under force, of the contents of the dog's stomach and/or small intestine.

URGENCY INDICATOR

Where the vomiting is severe and frequent, veterinary advice must be sought immediately. The underlying condition must be investigated and treated, rather than attempting to treat the symptom.

Underlying causes

Vomiting is often brought on by something extremely simple, such as a rapid change of diet, or motion sickness. Other causes may include heatstroke (see p. 114) or other conditions that affect the chemical composition of the blood, such as diabetes mellitus (see p. 28), renal failure (see p. 36), liver disease (see p. 94), or a bacterial infection. A foreign body in the stomach, gastric dilation/torsion or even stomach cancer would also cause vomiting, as would a heavy load of parasitic worms (see p. 71), constipation (see p. 35) or diarrhoea (see p. 32). Fear and stress, a trauma to the head or an infection such as canine parvovirus or canine distemper may also have vomiting as a symptom.

Owner action

If your dog suddenly and repeatedly vomits, prevent him from eating or drinking anything, and contact the vet. Keep the dog where you can see him, covering the floor with newspapers or similar to keep your home clean, and note the times of vomiting, and also the consistency, colour and quantity of the vomit. By doing this, you will help the vet to find the cause of the sudden vomiting, and thereby treat the problem effectively.

Occasional vomiting is normal, and no action need be taken in such cases. However, in cases of recurring vomiting, or where large amounts of vomit are being produced, or there is blood in the vomit, veterinary advice should be sought. Vomiting which you consider is a result of your dog's scavenging, and which is therefore spasmodic and not severe, is best treated by starving the dog for 24 hours. During this time, it is vital that the dog is offered regular small amounts of water to drink, to help prevent dehydration. After this time, re-introduce food with small light meals, such as scrambled eggs or boiled chicken, gradually building up to his former feeding regime. If the vomiting continues, or starts again when food is re-introduced, seek veterinary advice as soon as possible.

You can help prevent some of the causes of vomiting by ensuring that all your dog's vaccinations are kept up-to-date, treating him on a regular basis for internal parasites (worms), discouraging him from scavenging, not making sudden

⚙ **COST**

Depends on the underlying cause of the vomiting. For example, if vomiting is caused simply by dietary problems, the treatment will be simple and cheap, whereas if the vomiting is caused by diabetes mellitus (see p. 28), more veterinary treatment will be required, and the cost will be greater.

DIAGNOSING CAUSES OF VOMITING

The vet may need to carry out extensive physical examination, coupled with blood and other laboratory tests.

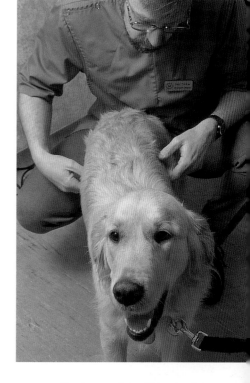

changes to his diet, not feeding him prior to travelling, and avoiding overfeeding.

Treatment
In severe cases, it is not unusual for the affected dog to be placed on an intra-venous drip to keep him hydrated. Where a foreign body is wedged in the animal's digestive system, surgery will be needed.

A physical examination by a vet will help ascertain the causes of your dog's flatulence, which is very often linked to his diet. Any change in this diet should be gradual.

Flatulence

Emission of gas from a dog's anus, often referred to as 'passing wind'.

Symptoms
A peculiar and often unpleasant smell around the dog, often combined with a characteristic noise.

Underlying causes
Flatulence may have several causes. If you feed your dog on poor quality food, he may not be able to digest it well before it passes into his large intestine, and it may begin to ferment; there may be chemical reactions within the dog's digestive system that are causing gases, or the gases may be a result of the dog bolting his food, and swallowing large amounts of air as a consequence. It may also be a symptom of serious digestive disorders, and so if the problem is persistent, it should be mentioned to the vet.

Owner action
If one particular food affects your dog by causing flatulence, change his food. It is a wise precaution to give your dog a good quality food, and avoid cheaper food of poor quality. A poor diet will have other detrimental affects on your dog, and will prevent him from becoming and staying fully fit.

Treatment
Normally, flatulence can be cured by changing the dog's diet, or simply avoiding feeding him the food(s) which cause the problem.

COST
Any changes to your dog's diet will be of relatively low cost.

Diarrhoea

Like vomiting, this is a symptom of another underlying condition and not an illness in itself.

Symptoms

Every reader will recognize the signs of diarrhoea. Greasy-looking feces and feces of different colours than usual are also classed as diarrhoea, as are small amounts of normal-looking feces that a dog passes very frequently, often having accidents around the home, despite being fully house-trained. If your dog is suffering from colitis, an inflammation of the colon (the first part of the large intestine), his feces will contain quite a lot of blood and mucus. This blood has an appearance totally different from the blood seen with internal bleeding. With internal bleeding, the blood will look dark brown and tarry, while with colitis, the blood will usually appear bright red. Another symptom of colitis is tenesmus, where the dog strains to defecate; this latter symptom is often mistaken for a symptom of constipation.

Underlying causes

Endoparasites, such as coccidia and whip worm are two of the most common causes of colitis in dogs, while stress and over-feeding are also prime suspects for diarrhoea. There can, of course, be many other possible causes – including foreign bodies in the digestive system and fungal infections – and the vet will need to carry out investigations before the condition can be treated effectively. There are some breeds that are thought to be more pre-disposed to colitis than others, but any dog can fall victim to this condition, and dogs of any age can be affected.

URGENCY INDICATOR

Diarrhoea causes the dog to dehydrate, and can lead to irreparable body damage (particularly of the kidneys) and even death. In all cases of severe diarrhoea, where over-eating is definitely not the cause, you should contact the vet. If the diarrhoea persists, or if there is blood in the motions, the vet must be consulted immediately.

DIAGNOSING CAUSES OF DIARRHOEA

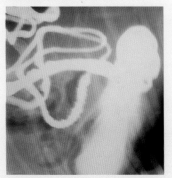

Laboratory analysis of samples of feces may be taken by the vet to ascertain the underlying cause of diarrhoea in your dog. If your dog suffers recurrent attacks of colitis, then X-rays and barium meals may be used to help find the best and most effective treatment for the condition.

Owner action

Prevent the dog from eating anything, but ensure that he is given adequate amounts of drinking water. If the diarrhoea is acute, provide the dog with a re-hydrating fluid, as described on p. 33. Contact the vet. Keep your dog where you can see him, covering the floor with newspapers or similar to keep your home clean, and note the times of his motions, and also the consistency, colour and quantity of the diarrhoea. By doing this, you will help the vet to find the cause of the sudden diarrhoea, and to treat the problem effectively.

The cause of diarrhoea may be a disease that can be transmitted to humans (zoonotic). Such diseases include campylobacter and salmonella, both caused by harmful bacteria. Take commonsense hygiene precautions to reduce the chance

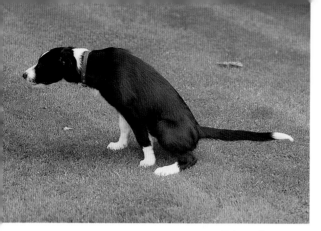

of any of these zoonotic diseases being passed on to you and your family. Always wash your hands after handling your dog, and particularly before eating. If you know that your dog has an infectious disease, you must make sure that everyone washes their hands after any contact with the affected animal.

Isolate the affected dog and keep him on water and electrolytes for 24 hours, dosing with kaolin solution (available from vets, doctors and pharmacies), about every two hours. After the fast, food intake should gradually be built up again; do not put the dog straight back on his original diet, otherwise the whole problem may recur. Chicken, rabbit and fish are excellent 'invalid' foods.

Treatment

The treatment for diarrhoea depends upon the underlying cause. If it is due to internal parasites, then anthelmintics (wormers) will be used to rid the dog of the infestation, while for infections, antibiotics will be used.

Endoparasites, stress and over-feeding are common causes of diarrhoea. If not treated this condition can lead to liver damage.

⊙ COST

Most cases of diarrhoea, especially those caused by simple dietary problems, will be cured at little cost. Barium meals and other such investigations will involve more veterinary care and treatment, so the cost will be considerably higher.

RELATED CONDITIONS WHICH MAY PRODUCE SIMILAR SYMPTOMS

Diarrhoea may be a symptom of more serious problems, such as enteritis (p. 34), which may result in feces that are both bulkier than normal, and also of a softer consistency. *ⓘ*

Cystitis

Inflammation of the bladder. It can affect both dogs and bitches.

Symptoms

These include urinating more frequently than usual, but often passing quite small amounts of urine, blood-tinged urine, or the animal showing severe discomfort when urinating. The urine produced may be foul-smelling, and the consistency may be thicker than normal. Cystitis is far more common in bitches than in male dogs.

Underlying causes

Most cases of cystitis are caused by a bacterial infection of the bladder from the genitals. Sometimes the cause is the presence of bladder stones.

Owner action

Feeding your dog slightly salted food will encourage him to drink more water than

---

URGENCY INDICATOR

Cystitis is not life-threatening, although it is often extremely distressing and painful for the affected animal. Veterinary treatment should therefore be sought as soon as possible.

DIAGNOSING CYSTITIS

A number of different bacteria may be the cause of cystitis, so a sample of urine from the affected dog will be required for the vet to diagnose and treat the condition accurately. ◉

Enteritis

usual. This regime should be combined with extra exercise to encourage more frequent urination. This will help to flush the urinary system through regularly.

Treatment
In straightforward cases of cystitis, the dog is usually treated with a course of antibiotics. The antibiotics must be given regularly, as directed by the vet, and the course must be finished for a full recovery.

Inflammation of the intestines, resulting in diarrhoea.

Symptoms
If your dog is suffering from diarrhoea, and shows signs of blood in his feces, this may be an indication of enteritis.

Underlying causes
Enteritis is very common among young dogs. It can be caused by different things but often it is the bacterium *Escherichia coli*, referred to as *E. coli*. Another major cause of enteritis is campylobacter bacteria; in humans, 'food poisoning' of this type is known as dysentery.

RELATED CONDITIONS WHICH MAY PRODUCE SIMILAR SYMPTOMS

Diabetes mellitus (see p. 28) is another possible cause of frequent urination, as is trauma of the bladder (usually caused in a road traffic accident, or similar accident) and bladder 'stones'.

A dog may develop stones in his or her urinary system (usually but not always in the bladder). These stones are known as uroliths, and the condition as urolithiasis; in severe case of urolithiasis, the male dog's urine flow may be completely blocked, and this could lead to acute renal (kidney) failure (see p. 94). Symptoms of urolithiasis include the passing, at more frequent than usual intervals, of often quite small amounts of urine, blood-tinged urine, the animal showing severe discomfort when urinating, incontinence, or the dog straining in the effort to pass urine. In the vast majority of cases of urolithiasis, the cause is a urine infection.

Urolithiasis is often treated by surgery, to remove the obstruction or to establish another opening through which the urine can be expelled. *i*

🖉 **HOMEOPATHIC TREATMENT:** Depending on the underlying causes of the condition, nux vomica, chimaphila or cantharis may be effective in the treatment of cystitis. Your vet will advise you further.

💧 **COST**
As most cases of cystitis can be cured easily in a very short time by a course of antibiotics, cost will be low.

DIAGNOSING ENTERITIS

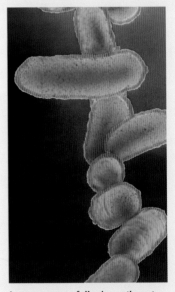

In many cases of diarrhoea, the vet will want to send samples of the dog's feces for laboratory analysis, to ensure effective treatment of the problem.

Constipation

Owner action

Observe your dog's actions, and the amount, colour, consistency and smell of your dog's motions. In particular, look for any signs of blood in the feces.

Treatment

Immediate treatment with a broad-spectrum antibiotic, together with regular doses of kaolin, may cure this condition. Sometimes more than one antibiotic will be needed, or even two or more courses of antibiotics.

URGENCY INDICATOR

Enteritis can be life-threatening, and treatment must be started as soon as possible.

COST

If caught early, a straightforward case of enteritis will be cured by a low-cost course of antibiotics, although the costs will obviously escalate if more treatment is needed.

RELATED CONDITIONS WHICH MAY PRODUCE SIMILAR SYMPTOMS

All dogs are potentially at risk from diarrhoea (see p. 32), with young dogs being more likely to suffer than adult dogs. In addition, some breeds, such as the German shepherd dog, are extremely prone to stomach upsets and diarrhoea, and many vets believe that these problems may be hereditary. In German shepherd dogs, one of the main causes of diarrhoea is a digestive disorder known as exocrine pancreatic insufficiency.

Failure by the dog to pass feces (or passing few and less frequently than usual). A symptom, not a disease, which may have many causes.

Symptoms

A dog producing extremely dry feces, or straining while (attempting to) defecate are all signs of constipation. Every dog (and its lifestyle) is different, but dogs should be expected to defecate between one and four times daily.

Underlying causes

Any debilitating disease can cause constipation, as can a foreign body blocking the dog's digestive system (usually in the intestines). In male dogs, an enlarged prostate gland is another possible cause (see p. 78).

DIAGNOSING CAUSES OF CONSTIPATION

A physical examination, particularly of the dog's rectum, will be necessary. In many cases, X-rays will also be taken to check that there is no physical blockage present.

Owner action

Regular exercise, a diet high in fibre and giving a good overall balanced diet will help prevent many cases of constipation.

Treatment

Where an internal blockage is the cause, the dog will need surgery. In cases linked with diet, laxatives and a change of diet may be all that is needed.

URGENCY INDICATOR

All of these conditions are potentially very dangerous, and so all cases of constipation must be taken seriously, and affected dogs referred to a vet.

COST

If surgery is needed, costs could be high.

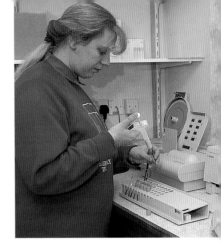

Renal failure

Failure of the kidneys. Waste products from digesting protein are removed from the dog's body by the kidneys; these two organs also regulate the body's water levels, and filter the blood to maintain the levels of various chemicals in the body fluids. They pass the waste products along to the bladder and through the nephrons in the form of urine. The nephrons are parts of the kidneys which remove various unwanted substances such as urea, uric acid and excess sodium from the blood.

URGENCY INDICATOR

Renal failure is life-threatening. Do not hesitate to contact the vet if you suspect this condition in your dog.

Symptoms

These include a seemingly insatiable thirst, the passing of large amounts of urine either in one go or at very frequent intervals, vomiting, diarrhoea, loss of appetite, weight loss, halitosis and anaemia.

Underlying causes

For various reasons, including infections and physical damage, the nephrons may fail to do their job properly, and this will lead to chronic renal failure. This is an extremely serious and usually irreversible condition with a very poor chance of recovery. The condition rarely occurs in dogs under the age of five years.

Owner action

Any dog showing signs of renal failure should immediately be taken for veterinary examination.

Treatment

Treatment of an affected dog may include a period of intensive care, during which the dog will have fluids administered via an intravenous drip, plus a special diet, coupled with a restful lifestyle and a prescribed course of medication. A dog suffering from renal failure will die, and you may choose to have your dog put to sleep.

DIAGNOSING RENAL FAILURE

The vet will arrange laboratory analysis of urine, X-rays and ultrasound examinations. These tests will look for signs that the kidneys are not working, that is the nephrons are not removing urea, uric acid and sodium from the blood plasma. 👁

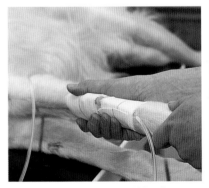

Renal failure is a serious condition, and it may be necessary for your dog to have fluids administered by intravenous drip.

🔋 COST

Due to the long-term nature of the intensive treatment required, veterinary costs will be high.

Urinary incontinence

The involuntary and uncontrolled passing of urine. This is far more common in bitches than in male dogs, particularly bitches that have been spayed.

Symptoms

If your bitch is constantly dribbling urine while lying down or sleeping, she may be affected by urinary incontinence, and will need to be examined by a vet. If a dog (male or female) dribbles urine when excited or exercising, this is a behavioural problem, not a medical one.

Underlying causes

There are many possible cause of urinary incontinence, which may include faulty urethral valves, congenital defects of the dog's urinary system, urolithiasis, cancer (see p. 98) or prostate problems (in male dogs – see p. 78).

It is much more common in bitches of medium to large breeds, and some breeds appear to be more susceptible to this condition than others.

Owner action

When taking your dog for veterinary examination, take along a fresh sample of the affected dog's urine.

It is unfair to punish or reproach a bitch for incontinence. Instead, you should make arrangements to enable her to relieve herself during the night.

A suitable bed for an incontinent bitch can be purchased, or one can be made easily from a large bean bag. These bags are commonly sold as dog beds, and older dogs love them. They support the dog's weight in an even fashion, and are warm and comfortable. In order that urine does not soak into the bag itself, leading to bad smells and becoming a health risk, waterproof the bag by placing it in a large heavy-duty polythene bag. This should then be covered with several thick layers of newspaper, and the whole thing covered with an old blanket or towel. If your bitch does have an accident in the night, the newspaper can be disposed of, and the blanket easily washed.

Treatment

Surgery may be needed to reposition an affected dog's bladder, while drug therapy may be used to improve the effectiveness of the urethra in sealing the flow of urine.

 HOMEOPATHIC TREATMENT: Depending on the underlying cause of the problem, low-potency oestrogen, causticum, gelsemium, turnera and ustilago can be effective. Consult your veterinary surgeon for further details of homeopathic treatment.

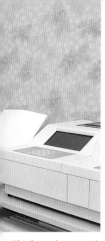
Blood samples, passed through a special machine, will help indicate any abnormalities which may be linked with renal failure.

URGENCY INDICATOR

Not life-threatening in itself, but as some of the possible underlying causes may be serious, it is much better to seek veterinary advice sooner rather than later.

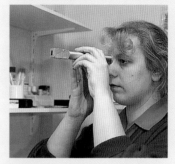
DIAGNOSING URINARY INCONTINENCE

Laboratory analysis of the affected dog's urine, X-rays and ultrasound may all be required to get a full and accurate diagnosis of the condition.

COST
This will vary enormously, depending on the underlying cause(s) of the condition.

Anal sac disease

Infection of the anal sacs. The dog has two anal sacs, just below the anus; one is at 8 o'clock and the other at 4 o'clock. They secrete an oily liquid, light brown in colour, that is expressed via two tubes as feces pass through the anus. It is thought that this liquid, which smells very bad to humans, is used as a means of recognition between packs and even individual dogs, and amounts are deposited along with every piece of feces passed by the dog.

Symptoms
In an effort to relieve his discomfort, an affected dog may take to licking the area around the anus, and this can cause further problems. A dog who licks at his infected anal glands will spread the

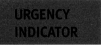

URGENCY INDICATOR

An uncomfortable condition for your dog, which should be relieved as soon as possible.

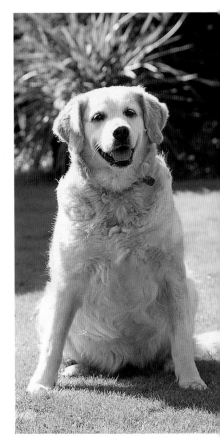

DIAGNOSING ANAL SAC DISEASE

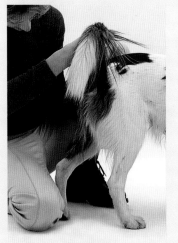

The vet will carry out a physical examination of the dog's rectum. ◉

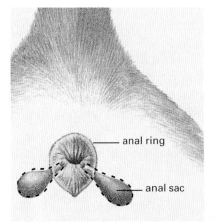

anal ring

anal sac

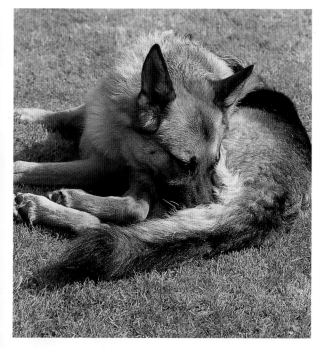

Above left: **A dog dragging his back end along the floor is another sign of anal sac disease.**

Above: **A dog which spends a lot of time licking the area around his anus may well be showing symptoms of anal sac disease, and should be examined by a vet.**

Left: **A cross-section of the anal region.**

infection to his mouth or throat, and this may lead to tonsillitis or pharyngitis (see p. 26). Where a dog is overweight, he may not be able to get to his anal glands, and so will be seen to nibble and lick at his flanks as he attempts to relieve the pain around his anus.

Other symptoms of anal sac disease include the dog chewing at one or more of his feet, dragging his back end along the floor, obvious swellings at the site of the anal sacs, and in cases where the sacs have become infected, ulcerated and burst, a mixture of blood, pus and foul-smelling brown liquid will be seen.

Underlying causes

When the liquid in the anal sacs becomes thicker, which may be due to an infection, it may become more difficult for the liquid

to be expressed, and this leads to a condition known as overfilling. If the dog starts producing the liquid at a faster rate, or the muscle tone around the anus alters, this can also lead to overfilling. The liquid in the overfilled sac then becomes impacted, and the sacs may become infected, causing the dog distress and pain.

It is impossible to know if a specific dog will suffer from anal sac problems, although smaller breeds seem to be more prone to this problem and, while many dogs never experience it, others suffer on a recurrent basis.

Owner action

If your dog shows any of the symptoms listed above, he should be taken for examination by the vet; if there is a discharge from the anal sacs he should be taken as soon as possible.

Treatment

If the problem is found to be overfilled anal sacs, the vet will empty them, which will ease the dog's discomfort. If the sacs are infected, then the dog may need to be given a general anaesthetic and have his sacs flushed out. Antibiotics will be given to a dog with infected anal sacs.

🕐 COST

Costs for treating simple overfilled sacs will be fairly low, although any necessary treatment for an infection of the sacs will add to the cost.

Movement

In mammals, movement (or locomotion) is brought about by the musculoskeletal system. This is made up of muscles, bones, ligaments, cartilage, tendons (which attach muscle to bones) and other supportive structures. The system also supports and protects the animal's vital organs.

In the dog, the forelimb is joined to the trunk of the animal not by a socket joint, but by muscles alone. This arrangement is ideal for an animal such as the dog, which has to run to live, as it gives a form of shock absorber, rather than the jarring which would result from a bony attachment. The hind limbs produce the main propulsion for the dog, so they are joined by a rigid bone called the pelvic girdle.

Normally, all of the dog's bones, muscles, ligaments, cartilage, tendons and other supportive structures work well together to keep the dog mobile. However, accidents can happen, and certain diseases will interfere with the workings of the musculoskeletal system. Any disorders, problems or ailments concerning the musculoskeletal system are likely to be extremely painful and disabling for the dog.

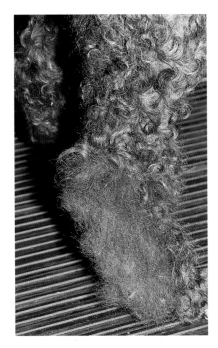

Feet covered with matted fur will be very uncomfortable for any dog, and the foot should be trimmed well before the problem reaches this stage.

Lameness

A dog is lame if he is incapable of normal locomotion, or he is moving with a gait that is not normal.

Symptoms
Hobbling or strange, painful and often laboured movement. The dog may be reluctant to put any weight on his affected leg, and that leg may be abnormal in appearance.

Underlying causes
Lameness may be caused by a variety of conditions but, in general, it is a symptom of pain in a limb or supporting tissues. Lameness may also be caused by deformities such as short limbs, or by the abnormal shortening of the muscles of the limbs.

Some causes of lameness are easily corrected, such as splinters in a foot, or a broken claw, while other types of lameness are caused simply by parts wearing out in an older dog (see arthritis p. 42).

Owner action

The first place to look for the cause of sudden mild lameness is the dog's paw. Examine it carefully for any obvious injury such as a cut or graze, a foreign body, balled fur, or a piece of grit; this is likely to be in one of the pads under the foot. If the injury is a small foreign body, such as a grass seed, it should be carefully removed with a pair of tweezers. The wound should then be cleaned with saline solution, and afterwards a little antiseptic ointment applied.

With long-haired dogs with hairy feet, such as English springer spaniels, the hair between the toes can ball up and make walking very uncomfortable for the dog. Any such hair should be gently trimmed off, using round-ended scissors to avoid stabbing the dog's foot if he moves. It is very useful to have someone to help when you are doing this.

During winter, your dog may pick up pieces of salt grit, which will have been spread on the road to help reduce the effects of frost, ice and snow. This grit has a nasty habit of getting into a dog's feet, making walking an extremely painful experience. After any walk in such conditions, examine your dog's feet. If there is evidence of salt grit in the feet, wash the affected feet in warm water. After washing, inspect the feet again, and apply antiseptic ointment on any area where the skin is inflamed or broken.

During the summer months, grass seeds are a potential problem for dogs, particularly active dogs who spend much

DIAGNOSING CAUSES OF LAMENESS

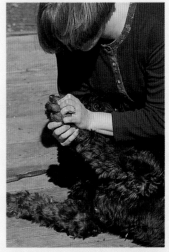

Physical examination of the affected feet or legs should be undertaken. The vet may need to use X-rays and other examinations to find the cause of any lameness.

time running in grassed fields and other areas. Grass seeds are particularly dangerous because their shape helps them 'worm' their way into the skin, but makes extraction very difficult.

Treatment

Where the lameness is only mild, but has suddenly appeared, it is likely that the problem is simple, and therefore easy to cure. Where the dog is suffering from acute lameness, the treatment will be entirely dependent on the underlying causes of the condition.

If a grass seed has entered the dog's skin, and it is not found, surgery may be necessary to remove it.

URGENCY INDICATOR

Very often lameness is progressive, and until the underlying cause is tackled, the problem will get worse. Cases of sudden and acute lameness, where the animal is completely unable to walk properly, must be referred to the vet as soon as possible.

COST

Mild lameness is usually simple to treat and therefore low cost, but other cases of lameness may involve quite complicated and expensive treatment such as surgery.

Arthritis

Inflammation of the joints. There are two forms of arthritis that commonly affect dogs – these are osteoarthritis and traumatic arthritis.

Symptoms
Swollen joints, difficulty in walking, lameness.

Underlying causes
Osteoarthritis may be a condition in itself, or a result of other conditions, such as hip dysplasia (see p. 50), while traumatic arthritis is caused as a direct result of an injury to the joint. Such injuries may be as a result of a road traffic accident (RTA), or a sprain while exercising.

Osteoarthritis is a progressive and very painful disease that will seriously undermine the quality of life of the dog. It may affect one or more joints, and the seriousness of the condition will depend on which joints are affected, and the general health of the dog. Overweight dogs are more likely to suffer from osteoarthritis.

Arthritis may be the result of poor nutrition, particularly in the early months of your dog's life, it may be hereditary, or it may be the result of poor husbandry and old age. The latter is almost always the case where a dog beyond middle age, who has been used to running and working in all kinds of weather, is given a kennel where he cannot keep sufficiently warm, and may even have to sleep on a cold floor without being able to get out of draughts.

Owner action
Careful exercise routines, detailed by the vet, will prove beneficial in may cases. Swimming is good, as it exercises the dog's muscles without putting pressure on affected joints.

DIAGNOSING ARTHRITIS

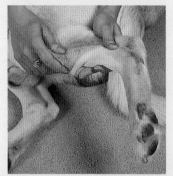

Physical examination and observation of the dog's movement will give the vet an indication of the problem. X-ray examination and analysis of samples of fluid taken from the affected joint(s) will often be necessary.

Treatment
The treatment for arthritis may include anti-inflammatory drugs and painkillers, a special carefully controlled exercise regime, and regular massages for the dog. In some cases, particularly where the osteoarthritis involves the dog's hips, your vet may recommend a hip replacement operation for the dog.

Spondylosis

A degenerative disease of the bones in the spine (vertebral column).

Symptoms
These include dragging of the feet and lack of coordination.

DIAGNOSING SPONDYLOSIS

The vet will confirm the diagnosis by X-ray examination (radiography).

COST
As no real treatment exists, the only costs involved will be for consulting the vet and the drugs to use to alleviate the pain and discomfort associated with the condition.

Underlying causes
Some dogs are genetically predisposed to spondylosis, and it is common in the larger breeds such as the Great Dane and Dobermann. It is usually seen when the dog is between eight and 12 months old, although it may also occur as a consequence of wear and tear, and so may be seen in elderly dogs.

Treatment
There is no cure for spondylosis; veterinary treatment will consist of trying to alleviate the pain and discomfort associated with the condition. It will not be necessary to have the dog put to sleep unless your vet considers that he is in too much pain.

Paralysis

Inability to move a limb or other part of the body, or loss of feeling in part(s) of the body.

DIAGNOSING CAUSES OF PARALYSIS

X-ray and ultrasound examinations may be used to determine the underlying cause of the paralysis.

Symptoms
Paralysis is a symptom of disruption of the nervous system. Affected muscles cannot work normally, and internal organs may be affected. Where a limb is affected, it is likely that the dog will drag this limb in an obvious fashion. However, where the paralysis affects internal organs, the symptoms may not

be so obvious, often simply manifesting themselves as the dog seeming 'off colour' or 'not himself'.

Underlying causes
Paralysis can be caused by any injury or trauma to the dog's brain, nerves or spine; road traffic accidents (RTAs) are a major cause of such injuries. Infectious diseases and infections may also bring on paralysis.

Owner action
Keep the dog calm and prevent any attempts at movement until a vet has carried out a thorough examination.

Treatment
The effectiveness of therapy will depend on the extent of the nervous injury and the time elapsed between the injury and the beginning of therapy. The type of therapy used will depend on the underlying cause of the condition.

RELATED CONDITIONS

Degenerative disc disease (see p. 44)

COST
There are many causes of paralysis, so the treatment costs will vary.

Degenerative disc disease

The breakdown (degeneration) of one or more of the discs down a dog's spine. The discs, known as intervertebral discs, separate each vertebra (piece of bone in the spine) and act to cushion and absorb shock, while forming joints that allow the vertebral column, or backbone, to bend and move. The discs themselves consist of a tough, fibrous outer band (known as the annulus fibrosus) which encases a jelly-like centre (known as the nucleus pulposus). The condition makes spinal injuries more common, and damage to the spinal cord is almost inevitable.

DIAGNOSING DEGENERATIVE DISC DISEASE

X-rays will usually pinpoint the exact location of the damage. Where they cannot, the vet may use a more specific test called a myelogram. A myelogram involves an injection of a dye, visible on X-ray examination, directly into the spinal column. This will not only show up the exact location of the problem, but also the amount of damage that has occurred to the disc itself.

Symptoms

The symptoms of degenerative disc disease vary depending on the severity and location of the problem. In milder cases, where there is only slight pressure on the spinal cord, the dog will be reluctant to move, even for toileting purposes or to eat his meals. If the dog does move, he may yelp or squeal when moving. Even if the dog does manage to move, he may appear to be uncoordinated and will stagger around, often tripping over his own feet, or he may not appear to have enough strength to walk properly.

Symptoms of complete ruptures are far more severe than those of partial ruptures. In severe cases, partial or even complete paralysis may occur. Sometimes only one limb appears to be affected, while in other cases, all four limbs are affected, injuries higher up the neck giving more severe symptoms. It is also quite common for paralysis in an affected dog to spread to the bladder, causing incontinence. Although ruptures can occur almost anywhere along the vertebral column, they are more likely to occur between the dog's pelvis and his last rib, or in the dog's neck.

Underlying causes

Degeneration is inevitable as a dog gets older, but may also be caused by the animal's lifestyle: a working dog or one that is extremely active will suffer more wear and tear on the discs than a lap dog.

It is the nucleus pulposus, the jelly-like centre of the disc, which acts as a shock absorber, that begins to degenerate, and the discs become less effective and less resilient. This leaves the disc(s) involved without a shock absorber, so even normal day-to-day activities may become very painful for the affected dog.

Where a dog is already suffering from degenerative disc disease (the owner may not even be aware of it), a sudden or severe trauma may trigger a reaction with the disc which leads to the nucleus pulposus of the disk being pushed into the spinal canal, causing severe damage of the spinal cord and its associated nerves. In severe cases, all that may be needed to trigger a rupture is a simple activity such

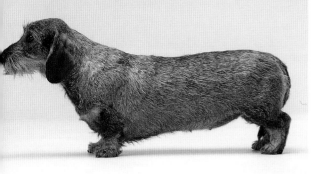

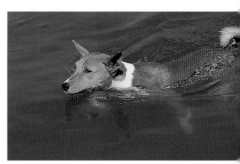

Above: **Dogs with long bodies, such as this dachshund, are extremely susceptible to degenerative disc disease, although any breed can suffer from this affliction, particularly if the dog is obese.**

Above right: **Many vets recommend using hydrotherapy or swimming to help dogs mildly afflicted with degenerative disc disease.**

as jumping off the sofa. Where the rupture into the spinal canal results in only a small amount of the nucleus pulposus entering the spinal canal, it is know as a partial rupture, whereas when the whole of the nucleus pulposus enters the spinal canal, it is known as a complete rupture.

An overweight dog of any breed (including crossbreeds or mongrels) has an increased risk of degenerative disc disease. Any dog can suffer from this condition, although dogs with long backs, such as the dachshund, are most likely to suffer, while other susceptible breeds include beagles, cocker spaniels, Lhasa Apsos, Pekinese and poodles. Symptoms may occur sooner in smaller breeds.

Owner action

Prevention is far better than cure, and there are some steps that you can take to help reduce the risk of your dog suffering from degenerative disc disease. Firstly, never allow your pet to become overweight, as this quite dramatically increases the risk of your dog having spinal (and many other medical) problems. If you own a breed that is known to be susceptible to spinal problems, you should try to discourage it from leaping and jumping, including on and off household furniture. Provide your dog with a bed of his own, and ensure that this is only very slightly raised from floor level. If you do not allow your dog to get on to your furniture from day one, he will never feel inclined to, and so you will prevent the problem arising.

Treatment

Severe symptoms indicate severe damage to the spinal cord, and the outlook for these cases is very poor, as treatment at this stage is rarely effective. In milder cases, once the problem has been diagnosed, and the exact location of the damage pinpointed, treatment can begin. The treatment will depend entirely on the extent of the rupture or damage to the disc. In very mild cases, a strict two-week period of confinement (usually, though not always, at the vet's surgery) is the beginning of the treatment. During this confinement period, the discomfort of movement helps to dissuade the affected dog from even attempting to move, thereby ensuring complete rest, and this prevents further damage to the affected disc(s). Twice daily physical therapy sessions follow, under strict veterinary supervision, and lasting about 15 minutes. Many vets like to use hydrotherapy (swimming) sessions, as this gives the dog exercise without putting undue pressure on the affected joints.

The vet may administer anti-inflammatory drugs during the dog's confinement period and, if necessary, conduct surgery to tackle the problem of the pressure placed on the spinal cord by the ruptured disc. This surgery is best carried out within 24 hours of the injury, and is known as a hemilaminectomy or a laminectomy.

With severely affected dogs, or where surgery has not been successful, many vets will recommend that the dog be humanely destroyed.

Fractures

Damage to bones caused by direct or indirect pressure. The bones may bend, split, crack, shatter or actually break. Where the bone is broken and pierces the skin, this is known as an open or compound fracture. Where there is one break that does not pierce the skin, it is a closed or simple fracture. Where a bone is broken into several pieces, the condition is known as a comminuted fracture. Any bones in the dog's body may fracture, although the most common fractures are those of the feet and legs.

Symptoms

Painful movement of the limb, tenderness, swelling, loss of control of the limb, deformity of the limb, unnatural movement of the limb, and crepitus (the sensation or, in very bad cases, the sound of the two ends of the bones grinding on each other).

DIAGNOSING FRACTURES

X-ray examination is almost always used to confirm fractures and also to discover the exact nature and extent of the fracture.

Underlying causes

Most fractures are caused by falls, road traffic accidents (RTAs), or where the dog has been kicked by a horse or similar animal. Puppies' bones are rather flexible, and can withstand quite major trauma without fracturing. However, where a dog has been fed a calcium-poor diet and the bones have not had the opportunity to grow strong, they will be very susceptible to fractures.

Owner action

Keep the dog quiet, and steady and support the injured limb, immobilizing it with bandages and splints if necessary, to prevent it moving and causing greater damage. Raising the limb will help reduce discomfort and swelling (by reducing the blood flow). Veterinary attention should be sought for every (suspected) fracture.

Treatment

Treatment depends on the extent and position of the fracture, but the aim is to allow the bone to mend itself. The first part of this process is to get the two broken ends to join, and then to prevent them from moving until the repair is healed. The most common method of holding the broken pieces of bone in place is by the use of casts and splints. In this method, once the broken ends have been manipulated back into the correct position, a rigid splint and/or plaster cast will be applied.

Surgery may be required to screw metal plates on to the pieces of bone, or in some cases just screws are used to keep the bone in place. One method that is common where long bones are involved, such as the main leg bones, is the use of long metal pins. Once the broken parts have been manipulated back into place, the pins are inserted down the centre of the bone, through the bone marrow. Wire is used to prevent any movement or twisting of the separate parts of the bone.

While many dogs will be allowed home within a few hours or days of surgery to repair fractures, others may have to spend a lot longer at the veterinary practice to ensure maximum care and effective treatment. Once your dog is back at home, you will probably need to administer prescribed painkillers and antibiotics (to

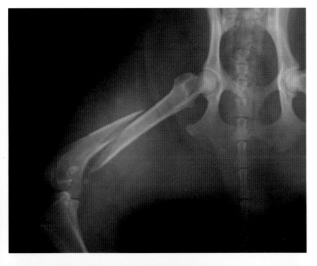

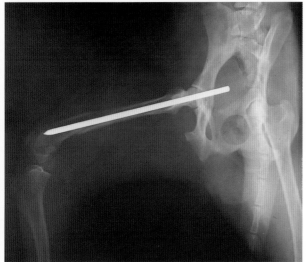

treat any infection), and perhaps to change dressings. It is important that you follow carefully the instructions that the vet gives you regarding medicines, feeding and movement. You will probably need to take the dog back to the vet for regular check-ups and, eventually, for the removal of casts, splints, screws or plates.

Whichever methods are used to repair fractures, the dog's rate of recovery will vary depending on several factors. Young dogs are likely to recover more quickly than older dogs, bones that have fractured into only two pieces will mend quicker than those with more breaks, while any infection will lengthen the whole process, regardless of any other factors that may be involved.

Top and left: **An X-ray of a fractured femur, before treatment ... and after. Note the pin which has been inserted down the centre of the femur to strengthen and support it until it heals.**

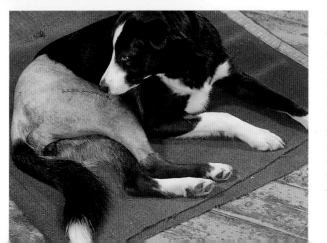

Where the fracture has been severe, it may be necessary to provide the dog with special nursing, until he is fit to be allowed home.

🕒 COST

Complicated and multiple fractures are likely to require pinning and in some cases more than one operation will be needed in order to carry out all of the work, thus adding to the overall cost.

Dislocation

The displacement of a bone from its joint.

Symptoms
Pain and swelling, loss of movement and paralysis. These symptoms are often accompanied by shock (see p. 116).

Underlying causes
Causes of dislocation can include bad falls, road traffic accidents (RTAs), fights, and even normal leaping and jumping. In some cases, notably dislocation of the hips, the cause is congenital, which means that the problem existed at birth, and is probably genetic in origin (see hip dysplasia p. 50). Trauma is another cause of dislocation of the hips, where the hips are perfectly normal prior to the trauma.

Owner action
If you suspect that your dog is suffering from a dislocation of a joint, you should keep the dog still and calm, and seek immediate veterinary attention.

Treatment
Treatment will usually consist of literally popping the joint back into its proper place. Although some dogs have this procedure carried out on them while they are conscious, most are sedated or anaesthetized. Painkillers will probably be prescribed. Rest leading to steady, easy exercise will help your dog to make a complete recovery.

URGENCY INDICATOR

In all cases of injury involving suspected dislocations of joints, urgent veterinary treatment should be sought.

COST

Unlikely to be too high in simple cases of dislocation of a joint, although any complications such as damaged ligaments can add to the cost of treatment, and often a dislocation is just one of the injuries sustained in a more serious accident.

Your dog may require further limb support after treatment from your vet.

DIAGNOSING DISLOCATIONS

X-ray and physical examinations will help the vet correctly diagnose the problem.

RELATED CONDITIONS

Fractures (see p. 46) and paralysis (see p. 43)

Poor exercise tolerance

Problems that make exercise difficult for the dog. With most breeds, it is often difficult to provide the dog with enough exercise, and this is particularly so with active working breeds such as English springer spaniels and Jack Russell terriers. Sometimes, however, a normally active dog will develop problems while exercising.

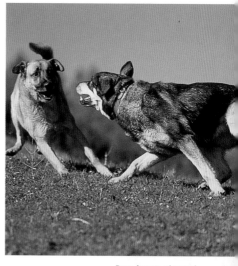

Dogs love to play and take exercise, and when this changes, it indicates a problem which will need to be investigated.

URGENCY INDICATOR

When a joint is damaged, the injury is referred to as a sprain, and may involve damage to cartilage and/or ligaments. While not dangerous in itself, the condition is painful. If not treated adequately, a sprain may eventually lead to osteoarthritis (see p. 42). Damage from osteoarthritis is usually permanent.

Symptoms
Pain and discomfort during what should be normal exercise.

Underlying causes
Often poor tolerance to exercise is a direct result of inflammation of the joints (arthritis – see p. 42), or malformation of the ball-and-socket joints, particularly of the hips (see hip dysplasia p. 50). Where a muscle is diseased (for instance with a bacterial infection), the term myopathy is used, and where a muscle is inflamed, the term myositis is used.

Owner action
Prevention is always better than cure. Ensure that your dog is dried properly before being kennelled. If the flooring is cold concrete, the dog's bed should be raised about 10 cm (4 in) off the floor, and he should be provided with some form of bedding.

Be very careful with regard to administering painkillers for sprains etc., unless under veterinary instruction.

Painkillers can easily lull a dog into a false sense of security, causing it to use injured joints which will result in more severe damage.

Treatment
In cases of mild myopathy, for example, where your dog develops a slight limp for 24–36 hours, simply resting him will probably relieve the problem, although if the limp persists beyond this time, veterinary advice and treatment should be sought.

🕒 COST
Sprains will cost very little in treatment costs.

DIAGNOSING CAUSES OF POOR EXERCISE TOLERANCE

Physical and X-ray examinations. 👁

RELATED CONDITIONS

Lameness (see p. 40), paralysis (see p. 43), hip dysplasia (see p. 50) and arthritis (see p. 42). ⓘ

Vertebral instability

Also known as wobbler's disease, this mainly affects the neck of the dog.

Symptoms
Affected dogs appear uncoordinated and weak, and may show signs of paralysis, although the dog will not appear to be suffering pain.

Underlying causes
Vertebral instability is caused by the fusing of the cervical vertebrae, and is mainly seen in Dobermanns and Great Danes, where the problem is thought to be hereditary. Any dog can suffer from the problem where it is caused by trauma.

Owner action
Keep the dog quiet and seek veterinary advice immediately.

Treatment
Anti-inflammatory drugs will be prescribed, and in many cases surgery will be required.

URGENCY INDICATOR

Veterinary advice should be sought as soon as possible.

◔ COST
If surgery is needed, this may involve more than one operation, and the costs will be high.

DIAGNOSING VERTEBRAL INSTABILITY

The vet will use X-rays to confirm the diagnosis. ◉

RELATED CONDITIONS

Paralysis (see p. 43). ❶

Hip dysplasia

Malformation of the hip joint. This complaint is particularly common in certain breeds (see below).

Symptoms
In dogs with distorted joints, normal use of the hip joints will result in varying degrees of inflammation and degeneration, causing the dog pain and suffering and making normal movements very difficult.

Underlying causes
Hip dysplasia is caused by a malformation of the hip joint. This poor fit means that the head of the femur (the ball) will rub on (and, over time, wear) the socket, causing severe pain and difficulty in walking for the affected dog. This development of the hip joint is especially crucial between 14 and 16 weeks, which is a particularly rapid growth phase in puppies.

While the main cause is undoubtedly genetic, poor nutrition in the early months of a dog's life can also predispose the dog to this condition. In breeds, such as Labradors and German shepherd dogs, where the disease is known to be hereditary, the breed societies urge breeders to have their dogs 'hip scored' before using them for breeding. Potential purchasers should check that the parents have good hip scores before finalizing any purchase of a puppy.

Owner action
Many governing bodies around the world run schemes to assess the degree of malformation in a dog's hips through X-rays. High scores are given to high degrees of hip dysplasia. All the scores for each breed are used to calculate an average for that breed, which are made available to breeders. Only dogs with hip scores well

URGENCY INDICATOR

Always take any dog showing symptoms of lameness to a vet at the earliest opportunity.

Many large breeds suffer from inherited hip dysplasia and should be 'hip scored' before being used for breeding purposes. This involves a vet taking X-rays of the dog's hips.

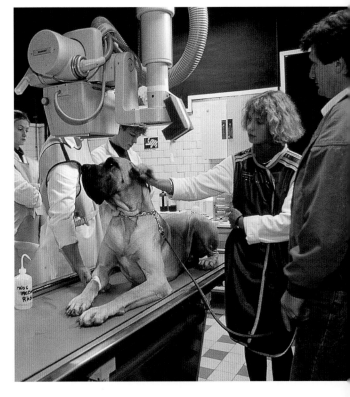

below the average should ever be used for breeding. When selecting a possible sire for a litter, breeders should look for those males who have produced offspring with low hip scores.

If you are considering using your dog for breeding, then you should make enquiries regarding having the dog's hips X-rayed. This can be carried out by your

DIAGNOSING HIP DYSPLASIA

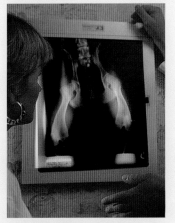

Both physical and radiographic examinations will be necessary to diagnose correctly the causes of hip dysplasia.

own vet, although as only the highest quality radiographs can be use for the scoring, your dog may have to be sedated or even anaesthetized, and this may mean that your dog is kept in the veterinary practice for up to a day.

Treatment

In mild cases, diet and gentle exercise (often accompanied by the administering of painkillers) may help the condition in the short term. However, the condition may eventually result in osteoarthritis (see p. 42), an extremely damaging condition. In older dogs, surgery may be called for, and this may include the reconstruction of the dog's pelvis or replacement of the hip joints.

🕐 COST

In all but mild cases, the cost of treatment for dogs affected with hip dysplasia is likely to be high.

Breathing and circulation

The respiratory system

Oxygen is supplied to the dog's body via the respiratory system. Air is breathed in through the mouth and nose and passes down the trachea or windpipe into the lungs, which are inside the chest cavity (thorax).

The windpipe consists of a tube lined with rings of cartilage, which help prevent the trachea from collapsing during normal breathing. The trachea passes into the thorax and then branches into smaller tubes, known as bronchi, which themselves branch, within the dog's lungs, into smaller tubes known as bronchioles. At the end of the bronchioles is a large number of alveoli, through which carbon dioxide is passed out of the body's system, while oxygen is taken in.

It is easy for small particles of debris, as well as airborne bacteria etc., to enter the respiratory system, but the cells lining the trachea and bronchi produce mucus, which helps to trap debris and airborne contaminants, stopping them from getting too far into the respiratory system. The airways also have tiny, finger-like projections, known as cilia. These cilia physically move away contaminants. The build-up of these contaminants, along with the mucus that has trapped them, results in coughing which expels the mucus and debris from the dog's body.

The respiratory system works together with the circulatory system, which is the body's blood supply. The blood supply to the lungs comes from the heart in an artery called the pulmonary artery. The lungs pass oxygen into the blood and the oxygenated blood is carried back into the heart. From there, the heart pumps the oxygenated blood around the body.

Without oxygen, or with insufficient oxygen, the dog's body would be unable to function, since oxygen forms the basis of all chemical reactions inside the dog's body. The dog's respiratory system has another, equally vital, role – the control of body temperature. Any problems with the dog's respiratory system can therefore have serious consequences for the dog's health.

Contagious respiratory disease
(Kennel cough)

Symptoms
A bad cough that worsens when the dog exerts himself, or pulls against the lead. The coughing bouts may end with the dog retching or gagging, and the cough sometimes produces mucus. There may be a discharge from the nose and a higher than normal temperature (a fever).

Underlying causes
A bacterium, *Bordetella bronchiseptica*, and also canine parainfluenza virus, either separately or together.

Owner action
Keep affected dogs isolated from others. It is normal for the condition to clear itself within a few days, and the dog should have made a complete recovery within 10–14 days. If it does not, you should seek veterinary advice.

HOMOEOPATHIC TREATMENT: Drosera or nux vomica for retching coughs. Dulcamara or stannum for a rattling cough. Coccus for coughs producing mucus.

COST Unlikely to be high, as little or no treatment is called for in most cases. It is only where secondary infections set in that costs may escalate.

Treatment
In severe cases, and depending on the underlying cause, treatment consists of antibiotics. Until recently, many vets also prescribed cough suppressants, but most modern vets consider cough suppressants to be of little use to an infected dog.

Dogs may be vaccinated against kennel cough. The vet sprays vaccine up the dog's nose, to stimulate the production of antibodies which will help fight off the infection. Such protection is essential if you are planning to send your dog to a boarding kennel.

DIAGNOSING CONTAGIOUS RESPIRATORY DISEASE

A physical examination, blood tests and tests of swabs from the dog's throat will be needed to identify the organism responsible for this condition.

URGENCY INDICATOR

Although not in itself too serious, kennel cough should be treated by a vet if the dog appears distressed by his coughing, or if he goes off his food. Even without any treatment, an infected dog will usually make a total recovery within 10–14 days, but prior vaccination is advised if your dog is likely to be exposed to any high-risk area, such as boarding kennels (hence the common name of the condition, 'kennel cough') or a dog show.

It is not unusual for a dog badly infected with contagious respiratory disease to suffer from lung damage if the condition is not treated.

RELATED CONDITIONS WHICH MAY PRODUCE SIMILAR SYMPTOMS

Breathing problems can be caused by a variety of conditions. Heart worms are parasites that live in the right-hand side of the heart and can clog up the pulmonary artery, reducing the blood flow to the lungs. The oxygen supply to the dog is therefore reduced, and breathing is difficult. Chronic bronchial disease (bronchitis, p. 54) is another possible condition that may cause similar symptoms.

Chronic bronchial disease
(Bronchitis)

Inflammation of the lining of the airways, leading to an excess of mucus being produced, which in turn reduces the space available in the airways for the passage of air. If this problem recurs, it can lead to permanent damage to the dog's respiratory system, in the same way as cigarette smoke and other pollution can damage the respiratory system of humans. Dogs kept by owners who smoke are more likely to suffer from bronchitis than those whose owners do not.

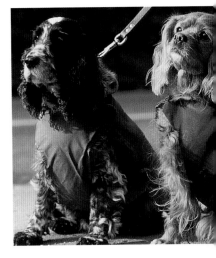

Smaller breeds of dog are prone to bronchial disease because of the small size of their respiratory system.

URGENCY INDICATOR

Never ignore any symptoms of a possible bronchial infection, even if mild. Seek veterinary advice.

☯ COST

In many cases of chronic bronchial disease, long-term therapy may be necessary, and this could prove expensive. Drug therapy may include medicines to suppress the production of mucus and antibiotics to control infection. Often it will be necessary for the vet to try out various combinations of drugs on the dog to find the best combination.

Symptoms
Persistent coughing, especially where mucus is coughed up by the dog. Rapid exhaustion, following or during normal exercise, and an increased breathing rate (a dog's normal breathing or respiratory rate is somewhere between 15 and 30 breaths per minute).

Underlying causes
Long-term exposure to polluted air is the usual cause. As the condition is of a long-term nature, older dogs (middle age onwards) are more prone to chronic bronchial disease. Small breeds of dogs are particularly susceptible to the condition, probably due to the small size of their respiratory system and the ease with which the airways can become clogged. Obesity also tends to make dogs more prone to this disease (as well as to many others).

Owner action
If your dog suffers from bronchitis, avoid taking him for walks in very cold conditions, as the cold air is likely to irritate his airways. You can help to relieve the dog's breathing problems by taking him into a steamy atmosphere, such as a bathroom where a large, hot bath has recently been run. The steam will reduce congestion.

Treatment
Any dog severely affected by chronic bronchial disease is likely to require long-term therapy. Treatment will normally consist of antibiotics to control any infection, along with drugs to reduce the production and build-up of mucus.

DIAGNOSING BRONCHITIS

Physical examination will normally diagnose the problem, followed by X-ray examinations and laboratory analysis of mucus and ◉

RELATED CONDITIONS WHICH MAY PRODUCE SIMILAR SYMPTOMS

Contagious respiratory disease (see p. 53). ⓘ

Rhinitis

Inflammation of the dog's nasal passages.

Symptoms

A discharge from the nose, together with bouts of sneezing.

Underlying causes

Bacterial or fungal infection can cause this condition. Where the discharge is from one nostril only (known as a unilateral discharge), this usually indicates a fungal infection, trauma or cancer. Where the discharge is from both nostrils (a bilateral discharge), this usually indicates a viral or bacterial infection. The fungus in question is usually *Aspergillus fumigatus,* also responsible for aspergillosis in birds and man. If *Aspergillus fumigatus* is responsible for your dog's rhinitis, the nasal discharge will be thick and green, and may persist for a long time – often months. Rhinitis can also be caused by foreign bodies trapped in the nasal cavity or a nasal tumour.

Owner action

Keep the dog calm, and do not allow him to exert himself. Seek veterinary advice as soon as possible.

Treatment

If the underlying problem is due to bacterial infection, the vet will prescribe a course of antibiotics. The whole course should be completed as directed. If the problem is caused by a blockage, surgery may be required to remove this. If a cancer is the cause, your vet will advise you on the best treatment. A fungal infection will be treated with anti-fungal drugs.

⊙ **COST**
If the condition can be treated by a simple course of antibiotics, costs will be low, but where surgery is necessary, costs will rise accordingly.

URGENCY INDICATOR

Veterinary advice should be sought if your dog shows any signs of this condition.

DIAGNOSING RHINITIS

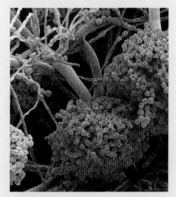

Laboratory analysis of the nasal discharge to diagnose the underlying problem. If a blockage is suspected, X-ray examinations will almost certainly be necessary, unless a physical examination finds the cause of the problem. ⊚

RELATED CONDITIONS WHICH MAY PRODUCE SIMILAR SYMPTOMS

Sinusitis, the inflammation of the mucous membranes in the nasal cavity, may produce similar symptoms. This condition can be treated with antibiotics. *ⓘ*

Collapsed trachea

This is a condition when the windpipe, a cylindrical tube lined with rings of tough material called cartilage, collapses.

Symptoms
Characteristic coughing, often described as similar to the honk of a goose, and distress during breathing (particularly when exercising) are symptoms of a collapsed trachea.

URGENCY INDICATOR

A collapsed trachea will adversely affect the breathing of the dog, and so urgent veterinary treatment must be sought.

DIAGNOSING A COLLAPSED TRACHEA

X-ray and endoscopic examination will help the vet diagnose this problem correctly, and determine its extent and severity.

Underlying causes
A collapsed trachea is caused by weakening of the interconnecting muscles of the cartilaginous rings that support the trachea. This weakening causes the trachea to collapse and flatten when the dog is breathing in or out, and it may be life-threatening as it can drastically reduce the dog's ability to breathe normally.

This condition is seen mainly in dogs aged six years and over, of the smaller (toy) breeds, particularly Yorkshire terriers and toy poodles.

Owner action
Try to make the dog as comfortable as possible, and keep him calm until veterinary treatment can be obtained.

Treatment
In all but very mild cases of collapsed trachea, surgery will be needed, and the problem can generally be corrected by the insertion of support rings, usually made from polypropylene or a similar material.

◔ COST
Surgery is almost always needed, and so costs could be quite high.

RELATED CONDITIONS WHICH MAY PRODUCE SIMILAR SYMPTOMS
Contagious respiratory disease (see p. 53) and chronic bronchial disease (see p. 54).

Pneumonia

Inflammation of the tissue on the inside of the lungs.

Symptoms

These include incessant coughing, coughing up quite large amounts of phlegm and mucus, difficulty in breathing, reluctance to take exercise or even move at all, fever, lethargy and lack of interest in food. A dog affected by pneumonia will typically stand with his front legs spread and head lowered, often coughing, but desperate to take in more air.

Underlying causes

Pneumonia can be caused by a bacterial or a viral infection, although not all cases of pneumonia are caused by this. Pneumonia can also be caused by the inhalation of food or vomit, smoke or even chemicals, and in these cases the affected dog is highly likely to suffer from secondary bacterial pneumonia.

Owner action

Keep your dog calm while veterinary treatment is sought. If there is a delay before the vet can see your dog, ensure that the dog takes in plenty of fluids. Most vets will appreciate the seriousness of the condition, and will see the dog quickly.

Treatment

As many body fluids are lost in the increased respiratory secretions in an affected dog, intravenous fluid therapy may be required. The vet may hospitalize your dog, and administer special drugs designed to expand the dog's airways, thus helping him to breathe.

Where the pneumonia is caused by inhalation or aspiration, it is almost impossible for a vet to remove the foreign substances, and it is highly unlikely that the dog will make a full recovery, often being afflicted with a cough for the rest of his life.

URGENCY INDICATOR

Urgent veterinary advice should be sought, as pneumonia is potentially life-threatening.

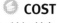 **COST**
Could be high, particularly if caused by inhalation of vomit or food, due to the subsequent infection. High doses of antibiotics and/or anti-fungal drugs will be needed, along with other drugs to open the airways, and intravenous fluids may need to be administered, all of which will add to the cost.

DIAGNOSING PNEUMONIA

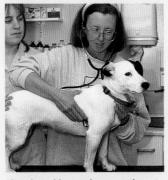

Listening with a stethoscope, the vet will be able to hear abnormal noises from the affected dog's lungs, although X-ray examination is needed to confirm a diagnosis of pneumonia. Blood tests from an affected dog will show higher than normal numbers of white blood cells, and often the vet will take a sample of fluid and mucus from the respiratory system in order to pinpoint the exact infection responsible. This will help to find the most effective antibiotic or anti-fungal to use in each case.

RELATED CONDITIONS WHICH MAY PRODUCE SIMILAR SYMPTOMS

Contagious respiratory disease (see p. 53) and chronic bronchial disease (see p. 54).

The circulatory system

The circulatory system is a series of tubes, running throughout the dog's body, through which blood circulates. The driving force for this circulatory system is the hear. Closely allied to the circulatory system is the lymphatic system, which carries the excess tissue fluid in the body, known as lymph.

There are two parts to the circulatory system – the pulmonary and the systemic. The pulmonary circulation moves deoxygenated blood from the heart to the lungs, where carbon dioxide is expelled from the body and oxygen is taken in. This oxygenated blood is returned to the heart, from where the systemic circulation takes it to tissue and organs around the body and returns deoxgenated blood to the heart.

Blood is carried away from the heart in large blood vessels called arteries that have thick, muscular walls. Within the organs, the arteries get smaller, and are known as arterioles, and within the tissues of these organs, the arterioles become even smaller, and are then known as capillaries. These blood vessels are very thin-walled, to allow exchange of gases.

Blood is carried to the heart in large, thin-walled blood vessels called veins. When such a vessel occurs within the tissue, to receive blood from the capillary bed, it is much smaller, and is known as a venule. Blood within veins is at much lower pressure than that within arteries.

The brain, the heart and the kidneys have a system of 'end arteries', capillaries that branch throughout the three organs, but do not join with one another. It is thought that these end arteries offer protection against sudden drops in blood pressure, as would occur after severe blood loss. At times of such loss, the dog's body will divert blood to these vital organs, as the other body organs are able to survive a period of restricted blood flow without suffering damage. If an end artery becomes blocked (for example, with a blood clot), blood flow is completely cut off, and the tissue will die. In the normal capillary bed, where a vessel becomes blocked, there are still many more routes through which blood can reach the tissues.

Blood itself serves many functions, including:
● transport of oxygen to the tissues;
● transport of carbon dioxide away from the tissues;
● transport of water to the tissues;
● thermo-regulation;
  assistance in the maintenance of the correct pH in the tissues (pH is the measure of acidity (low pH) or alkalinity (high pH) – a pH of 7 is neutral);
● transport of waste away from the tissues;
● transport of food to the tissues;
  blood- clotting to stop haemorrhaging;
● transport of hormones throughout the body;
● transport of enzymes throughout the body; and
● transport of antitoxins and antibodies throughout the body (to protect against infection).

The side view of a
dog's heart. The heart
is surrounded by lungs
and is protected by the
rib cage.

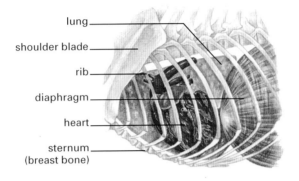

lung

shoulder blade

rib

diaphragm

heart

sternum
(breast bone)

The red colour of blood is due to the oxygen-rich haemoglobin – a protein containing iron – carried on the red blood cells. The white blood cells have the main task of protecting the body from infection. The other type of cells carried in the blood are the platelets, which help clot the blood, protecting against haemorrhage. Vitamin K is vital for this clotting, and certain rodent poisons (such as Warfarin) are designed to destroy vitamin K, thereby preventing blood clotting.

Heart problems

Heart disease is very common in dogs, and may lead to heart failure unless the problem is treated correctly. If the movement of blood through the heart is decreased for any reason, the dog's blood pressure will increase, and there may also be a build-up of fluid in the dog's lungs or abdomen. This can lead to congestive heart failure, depending which side of the heart has the problem. To help understand the potential problems, it is necessary to look closer at the heart and the way in which it should function.

The heart is a four-chambered, double pump in the centre of the thoracic cavity. Under normal circumstances, blood enters the heart's right atrium (top chamber) via the vena cava (a large vein), and is then pumped into the right ventricle (lower chamber), before being pumped via the pulmonary artery to the dog's lungs. Blood returning from the lungs enters the heart's left atrium via the pulmonary veins, and is then pumped into the left ventricle, from where it leaves, via the aorta (a large artery), to begin its journey around the dog's body.

The atria and ventricles are separated by valves (atrio-ventricular valves), which prevent the blood from flowing in the wrong direction. Where one or more atrio-ventricular valves are defective or diseased, there is a back-flow of blood, and this causes 'heart murmurs'.

Mitral insufficiency

A problem with the left atrio-ventricular valve leads to a condition known as mitral insufficiency.

Symptoms
Fluid build-up in the lungs, causing the dog to get out of breath very easily. The dog may have bouts of coughing, especially after exercise and also at night. His abdomen may become distended, and he may lose weight.

Underlying causes
If the left atrio-ventricular valve does not close correctly, it allows blood to flow from the left ventricle to the left atrium. This causes a reduction in the amount of blood pushed forwards by the heart, so the heart has to work harder to try to make up this deficit. At the same time, as blood from the lungs cannot get through the heart at the correct rate, a build-up of fluid occurs within the lungs. This leads to a drastic reduction in gaseous exchange in the lungs, which makes the heart try to pump more blood through the lungs and thus a dangerous cycle develops, leading ultimately to heart failure. Smaller breeds seem to be genetically predisposed to this condition.

Although the usual cause of mitral insufficiency is old age, normal day to day wear and tear having a damaging effect on the left atrio-ventricular valve, there can be another cause. Bacteria from diseased teeth and gums that enter the dog's bloodstream can damage the heart valve through infection or inflammation, and even when the infection and inflammation has cleared up, the valve may still be scarred and unable to carry out its work efficiently.

Owner action
Keep the dog calm, and do not allow him to over-exert himself.

Treatment
The condition is not reversible. Any treatment given can only relieve the symptoms, and prevent the condition from worsening. Diet may help to reduce fluid retention, and diuretics (drugs designed to increase the production and excretion of urine) may also be prescribed. Drugs may be given to dilate the blood vessels, making the heart's work slightly easier.

DIAGNOSING MITRAL INSUFFICIENCY

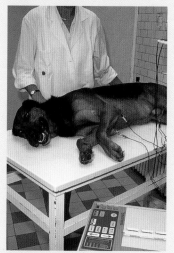

Physical examination using a stethoscope (listening for heart murmurs), followed by X-ray examination and electrocardiograms.

Cardiomyopathy

Disease of the heart muscle.

Symptoms

Fluid build-up in the lungs, causing the dog to get out of breath very easily. The dog may have bouts of coughing, especially after exercise and also at night. His abdomen may become extended, and he may lose weight.

This disease can lead to the enlargement of the dog's heart. There are two possible effects of this condition: one is the thickening and abnormal enlargement of the heart muscle, and is known as hypertrophic cardiomyopathy. The other is thinning of the wall of the heart, and this is known as dilative cardiomyopathy.

Both hypertrophic cardiomyopathy and dilative cardiomyopathy affect the ability of the heart to contract properly, causing symptoms very similar to those involving inefficient valves (see pp. 61 and 62).

Underlying causes

Very often, hereditary or congenital defects are to blame. The diseases are more common in the larger dog breeds.

Owner action

Keep the dog calm, and do not allow him to exert himself.

Treatment

If these problems are detected early in life, it may be possible to correct them by surgery, although this is only possible in a very small number of cases. Where the conditions are left for longer, they will cause heart disease.

DIAGNOSING CARDIOMYOPATHY

Using a stethoscope, the vet will listen for unusual (fast) heart rates, rhythms and murmurs. Radiographic tests (X-rays) will show any abnormality in the shape of the heart muscle. 👁

RELATED CONDITIONS WHICH MAY PRODUCE SIMILAR SYMPTOMS

Certain diseases, such as canine parvovirus in very young puppies, can affect the heart's function. It is also possible that a puppy could have a congenital heart defect. Such problems as valvular stenosis (problems involving the heart's valves), septal defects (affecting the wall of the heart) and patent ductus arteriosus (defects of the vessels leaving the heart) have all been seen in puppies. Mitral insufficiency (see p. 60) may also cause similar symptoms. ⓘ

Other heart problems

Symptoms

A dog suffering from a failing heart will show certain clinical signs of the problem. Early on, these signs are liable to be subtle, so it is wise to keep a wary eye on your dog. The symptoms that an affected dog may show include breathing difficulties, coughing (especially after exercise or at night), weight loss, exercise intolerance and a distended abdomen. A dog affected by heart problems may stand with his front legs spread and head lowered, often coughing, but also desperate to take in more air.

Underlying causes

There can be many causes of heart disease, some of which are congenital, such as faulty valves or a 'hole in the heart'. Heart muscle diseases and diseases of the tissues around the heart can also cause problems for the affected dog.

Owner action

Keep the dog quiet and calm, and arrange for someone to accompany you (or even better, to drive you) when you take your dog for examination by the vet.

Treatment

It is a sad fact that most cases of heart disease are not reversible, and any treatment merely makes the dog's condition easier to live with, rather than providing a cure. A slowing in the progression of the disease is the main aim of the vet in these cases.

To help reduce blood pressure and the amount of fluid in the heart or lungs, dogs with heart problems are fed on a special low-sodium diet. To reduce the build-up of fluid further, affected dogs are put onto diuretics, to increase the amount of urine passed. If your dog is put on diuretics, ensure that he always has plenty of water to drink, as his thirst will increase dramatically with these drugs.

These two treatments often result in a lessening of – or even complete relief from – the coughing and discomfort associated with heart disease. If they do not, then the vet may prescribe drugs to make the work of the heart easier, by dilating the blood vessels. If even this does not work, the drug digitalis may be given. This will help slow the heart's beat, while strengthening its contractions.

DIAGNOSING HEART DISEASE

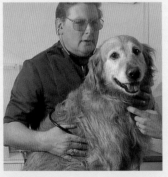

As most forms of heart disease are accompanied by heart murmurs, the vet will use a stethoscope to detect these, often before any other type of examination. Using his skill and training, the vet will be able to use a stethoscope to pinpoint the problem, from the position of the murmur to whether it occurs on the heart's relaxation phase, its contraction phase or both. The vet may also use X-rays and electrocardiograms to diagnose the exact problem. ◉

Anaemia

An overall reduction in the number of red blood cells in a dog's body, resulting in a lack of iron. This leads to the dog's cells not being supplied with sufficient oxygen for respiration.

Symptoms

These include an increased breathing rate, an increased heart rate, tiredness, weakness and pale mucous membranes, such as the gums.

URGENCY INDICATOR

As the underlying cause of anaemia could be serious, you should obtain veterinary advice as soon as you believe that your dog is suffering from this condition.

Underlying causes

There are many causes of anaemia. These may include:
kidney disease (see p. 36);
iron deficiency;
vitamin B12 deficiency;
hypothyroidism (a deficiency in the action of the thyroid gland, which produces the hormone thyroxin. This can lead to alopecia (see p. 65), weight gain, fatigue and cold intolerance);
cancer;
poisoning;
liver disease (see p. 94);
blood loss;
hookworms;
external parasites such as fleas, ticks and lice; or
gastric ulcers.

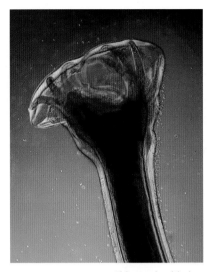

Ticks may be picked up when your dog is exercising, particularly in long grass. Examine the dog after such exercise, and remove any ticks.

DIAGNOSING ANAEMIA

Diagnosis will involve the vet taking blood samples for laboratory analysis, which will be able to detect the underlying cause(s).

Owner action

As this condition can only be diagnosed by a vet, the owner can do nothing other than seek veterinary advice.

COST

In severe cases, where much treatment is necessary, often including blood transfusions and other expensive treatments, costs are likely to be high.

Treatment

Treatment will depend upon the cause of the problem. It may be necessary for your dog to be given blood transfusions and oxygen therapy, which is the supply of pure oxygen, via a mask or an oxygen tent, to the affected dog.

The skin

The dog's body is covered by a protective layer of skin. Skin serves a number of functions:

- **it keeps out foreign bodies;**
- **keeps in moisture;**
- **regulates body temperature;**
- **manufactures vitamin D; and**
- **hair and skin pigment protects against ultraviolet radiation.**

It also contains sweat glands and receptors for pain, temperature and pressure. The skin is composed of three layers, the epidermis being the outermost layer, the dermis below that and the hypodermis being the innermost layer.

A dog's hair is actually formed from epidermis. It grows through a tube called the hair follicle. For each hair follicle there is a sebaceous gland, which lubricates and waterproofs the hair and skin. These glands produce a scent that the dog uses as a marker for its territory. They also produce hormones called pheromones that help attract members of the opposite sex.

- **There are three types of hair:**

  1. Guard hairs: the long hairs of the top layer of the dog's coat, which provide the waterproofing of the dog's coat.

  2. Undercoat or wool hairs: these trap air to keep the dog warm, and make up most of the coat of a puppy.

  3. Vibrissae: hairs that are sensitive to touch, the 'whiskers' around the mouth and eyes, and on each cheek.

NEVER CUT THE VIBRISSAE WITHOUT GOOD REASON.

Moulting is when the dog sheds his hair each season to have a coat suitable for that season: a thick winter coat and a thinner summer one. Sometimes larger than normal amounts of hair are lost; this is quite common, and it often leads to sections of the dog's body, usually his flanks, being almost totally without hair. The hair will usually grow back at the time of the next moult.

WARNING: MANY OF THE SKIN CONDITIONS WHICH MAY AFFECT YOUR DOG ARE ZOONOTIC, AND SO COULD ALSO AFFECT YOU.

Alopecia

Abnormal hair loss.

Symptoms
Loss of hair, which may be in small, localized patches or cover large areas of the dog's body.

Underlying causes
It is thought that stress can cause hair loss in dogs, as well as in humans. In bitches, this is most evident when the dog is pregnant or raising a litter of pups, and therefore lactating, when she is likely to lose much of her hair. In cases such as this, the hair almost always re-grows to its normal condition.

When fleas bite a dog to feed on his blood, they secrete saliva to prevent the blood from clotting, and some dogs develop an allergy to this saliva. This affliction is referred to as 'flea allergic dermatitis', and will cause the dog to scratch himself even more than he would do for a normal flea infestation. This leads to hair loss, often over a large part of the dog's body, in particular the flanks, tail and rump. This condition may lead to another skin condition – folliculitis, caused by a bacterium, and this may further intensify the problem. See pp. 66–71 for information on fleas and other parasites.

Owner action
As some skin complaints that cause alopecia may be zoonotic (that is, may cross to humans), care should be taken that you do not catch them. Common-sense hygiene precautions and practices should be followed. Always ensure that you wash your hands thoroughly with top quality soap after touching your pet. If you have reason to suspect that the problem is zoonotic, it is wise to wear disposable latex gloves whenever you handle your dog. Children in particular must be encouraged to carry out these hygiene routines.

Treatment
This depends entirely upon the underlying cause. If the problem is caused by ectoparasites, then a shampoo or ointment will be used. Open and sore areas of the dog's skin will need to be treated with antiseptic medicines.

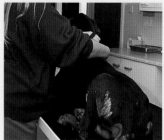

DIAGNOSING ALOPECIA

For accurate diagnosis of skin complaints, the vet will need to take 'skin scrapes' for laboratory analysis. The vet scrapes a small amount of the surface layers of the skin, and this skin sample is then examined under a microscope, where the vet or technician looks for telltale signs of the problem, such as parasites or their droppings.

RELATED CONDITIONS WHICH MAY PRODUCE SIMILAR SYMPTOMS

Many skin complaints will exhibit similar symptoms, so it is essential to obtain veterinary advice and guidance in all cases. Do not try to treat the condition with medicines obtained from a pet shop without a definite diagnosis, as these may result in the condition lasting longer and cause the dog more suffering. ⓘ

Fleas

Fleas are insects that live as parasites on other animals. Even the most pampered dogs can suffer from the unwanted attentions of parasites, these being either internal (endoparasites) or external (ectoparasites).

Symptoms

Fleas are the most common ectoparasite; they bite their host and then feed on the blood that appears at the bite site. This area will show an inflammatory reaction, and will cause a certain amount of irritation to the dog.

Underlying causes

By far the most common flea to infect dogs is the 'cat flea' (*Ctenocephalides felis*), although they may be infected with the dog flea (*Ctenocephalides canis*) if they are not in contact with cats. Dogs are also liable to infestations of the rabbit flea (*Spilopsyllus cuniculi*) and the hedge-hog flea (*Archaeopsylla erinacei*). Rabbit fleas group together around the ear, and hedgehog fleas are very large in comparison to the other types of fleas that your dog may catch.

Owner action

In all cases of flea infestation, all the dog's bedding must be removed and treated, as must the household carpets treated, along with other household pets, in order to break the life cycle of the flea. If you are only treating the affected dog(s), the you are not treating the whole problem. Treatment of the household will prevent flea eggs hatching, and the larvae developing.

Use anti-flea preparations to treat all bedding and the dog's bed itself. Do *not* use such powders and sprays where a bitch is still feeding her pups, as there is a danger of poisoning the litter.

Treatment

There are many insecticidal preparations available from the vet, in the form of sprays, powders, impregnated collars, or shampoos. The vet may suggest a natural remedy, such as a herbal preparation, or a collar impregnated with such a preparation. In the USA, diatomaceous earth (the fossilized remains of a single-celled alga) is popular as a flea treatment. It is dusted on affected dogs and also on carpets, rugs, furniture, pet beds and bedding, and anywhere that fleas and/or their eggs may collect. This material is entirely safe for humans and pets, but is deadly to fleas and many other insects, even at their larval stage. It works by the fine particles in the diatomaceous earth attacking the wax coating that covers the exoskeleton of the fleas, so that the affected fleas dry out and die.

DIAGNOSING PARASITE INFESTATION

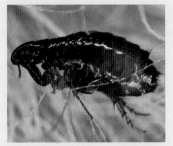

The vet will examine the fleas on your dog under a microscope. Identification of the flea can be carried out by the appearance of the flea's head, where the presence or otherwise of 'combs' is used to identify the particular species.

Mites

Mites are insect ectoparasites that have unpleasant effects on dogs, causing mange. There are three types commonly found: *Sarcoptes scabiei*, *Demodex folliculorum* and *Otodectes cynotis*.

Symptoms

The first sign of mange is persistent scratching, even though there is no obvious cause such as fleas. Eventually, the skin will become very red and sore, a symptom that is easier to see in the white areas of a dog's coat. As the disease progresses, these sores cause baldness and the sores themselves become worse.

Underlying causes

Sarcoptes scabiei is invisible to the naked eye and causes sarcoptic mange in dogs, leading to alopecia (see p. 65) and pruritus (intense itching), especially on elbows, hocks and ear flaps. *Demodex folliculorum* is a microscopic mite which is almost always present in the dog's hair, but only causes problems if its numbers increase, when it causes severe dermatitis and alopecia. *Otodectes cynotis* is a white mite that can be seen with a hand-held magnifying lens. This mite is almost always present in the ears of cats, where it causes no problems, but if it occurs in the ears of dogs it causes ear canker (otitis, see p. 12).

Dogs can become infected through coming into direct contact with other infected animals, such as rodents, or simply by being on infected ground. Mange is very common in dogs.

Owner action

Be warned – mange can be contracted by humans (in people, the condition is known as scabies). Take commonsense

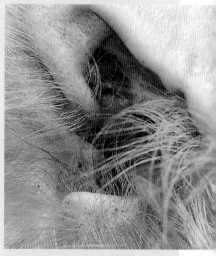

DIAGNOSING MANGE

Physical examination of the dog will be followed by microscopic examination of the mites found.

precautions to ensure that neither you nor your family will contract scabies, such as washing your hands after handling any dog that is believed to be infected with mites, or, even better, using disposable latex gloves.

Treatment

A wash that kills parasites must be applied to the affected areas. Use the wash under veterinary advice only. The dog's living quarters must be thoroughly treated by soaking in a strong solution of disinfectant or bleach, which must be washed off before any dog is returned to the kennel. Veterinary drug companies are continually producing new topical applications for this problem; your vet will be able to advise you on the availability and effectiveness of these products.

URGENCY INDICATOR

Mite infestations are best tackled as soon as they are noticed, to help prevent any complications.

◎ COST

If caught in the early stages of an infection, costs will be low. As the condition becomes more severe, it will become more difficult to treat, so the costs will rise accordingly.

Ticks

Like the flea, ticks are insect ectoparasites. By far the most common types of tick to affect dogs in the UK are the sheep tick (*Ixodes ricinus*), and the hedgehog tick (*Ixodes hexagonus*).

Symptoms
The dog will spend more time scratching itself, and you will be able to see the ticks, which look like small brownish-white or red-brown peas. They have their heads tucked under the top layer of the dog's skin.

Underlying causes
Ticks are ectoparasites that most dogs will catch at some stage. They are carriers of certain bacteria, harmful to many animals, and they also carry a range of diseases, such as Lyme's disease. Ticks may be contracted from other dogs, or from

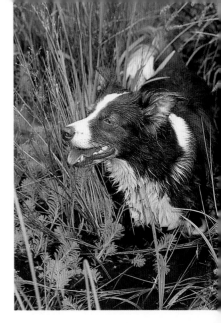

URGENCY INDICATOR

Ticks can cause irritation to the dog, and may move to humans. They are also capable of transmitting zoonotic diseases such as Lyme's disease. Therefore, you should obtain veterinary treatment for any dog carrying ticks as soon as possible.

DIAGNOSING TICK INFESTATION

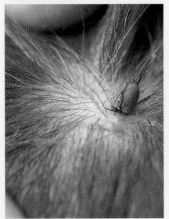

Physical examination of the dog's coat will reveal the ticks, which may then be identified.

other animal species including cats and rabbits. Both dogs and humans can pick up ticks as they brush against vegetation that is infested with these parasites. These ticks can cause irritation and itchiness, and anaemia in humans, while in the USA and Australia some ticks can cause paralysis.

Owner action
When an infestation of ticks has been discovered on your dog, all his bedding must be removed, and preferably burned, and the kennel thoroughly disinfected. Use 'tick powder', available from the vet, to treat all bedding and even the kennel or bed. Do *not* use such powders and sprays where a bitch is still feeding her puppies, unless the vet gives absolute assurances that it is suitable for this kind of use. With

Left: **Ticks may be picked up when your dog is exercising, particularly in long grass. It is important that you examine the dog after such exercise, and remove any ticks.**

Right: **Vets and pet shops sell tick removers which are specifically designed to remove the whole tick, without leaving the mouth parts still in the dog's flesh.**

Below: **A tick, greatly magnified. To the naked eye, they look rather like large, browny-white grains of rice.**

most of these powders, there is a danger of poisoning the litter as the powder attaches itself to the hair and even the nipples of the dam. The powders are designed for external use only, so can poison the pup if swallowed.

Treatment

Ticks are rather more difficult to deal with than fleas, but they do respond to some sprays and powders. In some countries, these may only be available from vets as they are classed as 'prescription only medicines', whereas in other countries they are freely available at pharmacies and even off the shelf in pet shops. The

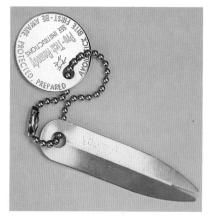

use of organophosphates, compounds found in flea and tick powders, on domestic animals such as dogs is banned in many countries.

Ticks attach themselves to their host by burying their head under the top layers of the host's skin, and use their mouthparts to feed from the host. Care must be taken when removing ticks to ensure that the mouthparts are completely removed from the dog's skin, otherwise infection and abscesses can occur; never simply pull ticks out. Paint alcohol on the tick using a fine paint brush, and the tick should have died and dropped off within 24 hours; if not, simply repeat the process.

Although some authorities suggest that ticks be burned off with a lighted cigarette, this should never be attempted. It is all too easy to burn the dog with the cigarette and the alcohol method is much more effective, with none of the dangers.

A number of devices are now on the market that have been specifically designed to remove ticks, due mainly to concern regarding Lyme's disease in humans. Among these is a type of sprung forceps that grip the tick around the head; the device is then gently twisted backwards and forwards until the tick comes out. I have tested several such implements and have had 100 per cent success with each; I now always keep one in my kennel first aid kit.

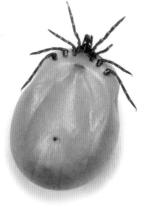

🔵 **COST**

Even the most modern and effective tick treatments are fairly low in price.

RELATED CONDITIONS WHICH MAY PRODUCE SIMILAR SYMPTOMS

Owners may mistake warts and other growths for ticks, or vice versa. ⓘ

Food allergies

Dogs may develop an allergy to one or more of the contents of their feed. Itchy skin will be a symptom.

Symptoms

Every animal (including humans) has the occasional scratch, but if your dog spends considerable lengths of time scratching at his coat, then you should seek veterinary advice.

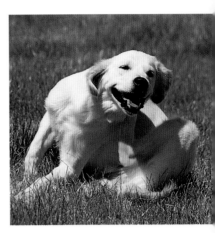

A dog which seems to be perpetually scratching itself may be showing symptoms of a food allergy.

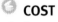 **COST**

It is often very difficult and time-consuming to find the food constituent(s) responsible for allergic reactions, and this will involve the vet's time which he will charge for.

URGENCY INDICATOR

It may be some time before the owner of an affected dog realizes that there is a pattern to the dog's problem, that is, the condition is linked with certain foods. Once this pattern emerges, the food(s) responsible for the allergic reaction should not be fed, and veterinary advice should be sought.

Underlying causes

Food allergies are caused by one or more of the contents of the feed, and there is much debate and controversy around the subject. Cow's milk, wheat and even some meats have been known to cause allergies in dogs and other domestic animals.

Owner action

Always feed a top quality diet, and only change it if necessary. Changing the diet should be done gradually over a period of seven to ten days.

Treatment

In many cases, the vet will need to take a blood or skin sample from the affected dog. The taking of a skin sample is an uncomfortable, though not painful, experience for the dog, in which the vet will use a scalpel to scrape a small amount of the surface layer of skin off the dog's body. This sample will then be sent for laboratory analysis, in order to identify the cause of the dog's condition. The laboratory procedures will include microscopic examination, in order to eliminate or confirm the possibility of mites or a fungal infection, such as ringworm (see p. 71).

DIAGNOSING ALLERGIES

Skin scrapes and blood tests may be needed. In some cases, the dog is put on a strict diet, with different food constituents being fed at different times, in order to find out which constituent(s) cause the problem.

RELATED CONDITIONS WHICH MAY PRODUCE SIMILAR SYMPTOMS

Ringworm (see p. 71), mites (see p. 67), fleas (see p. 66) and alopecia (see p. 65).

Ringworm

A fungal infection of the dog's epidermis and the hair fibres in the skin, and not, as some people believe, an actual worm.

Symptoms
The affected dog may spend time scratching himself, or rubbing against solid objects. There will be round areas of hair loss.

Underlying causes
The most fungi that are most commonly responsible for ringworm in dogs are *Microsporum canis*, *Microsporum gypseum* and *Trichophyton mentagrophytes*. The spores of these fungi may be wind-borne or found in the soil. All three types are highly infectious.

URGENCY INDICATOR

The condition is highly infectious, so veterinary treatment should be sought in all cases.

Owner action
Some of the fungi that can cause ring-worm are zoonotic. Care must be taken to ensure that neither you nor your family become infected, which can occur if you are in direct contact with affected areas of the dog's skin, or even if you are close to the animal if the spores are wind-borne.

Treatment
Ringworm is usually treated by washing the animal in a fungicidal wash prescribed by the vet, such as enilconazole. In some cases, the vet may 'paint' the affected areas with tincture of iodine, or apply an ointment (Whitfield's ointment), which consists of salicylic and benzoic acid and kills the fungus and prevents its spores escaping into the environment. All topical treatments (those applied directly onto the affected area) must be repeated for a full cure.

HOMEOPATHIC TREATMENT: Depending upon the actual organism responsible for the condition, bacillinium, berberis, chrysarobinum, sepia or tellurium may be effective. Ask the vet for advice.

COST The ointments and other medicines used to cure ringworm are low-cost treatments.

DIAGNOSING RINGWORM

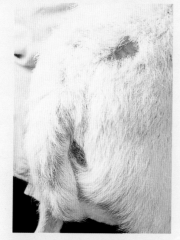

Ringworm appears as small round areas of hair loss. If these are looked at carefully, it is often possible to see the fungus around the edges of the affected area, often as whitish, scaly skin.

RELATED CONDITIONS WHICH MAY PRODUCE SIMILAR SYMPTOMS

Fleas (see p. 66) and alopecia (see p. 65).

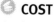

Pyoderma

Bacterial infection of a dog's skin.

Symptoms

These vary depending on the underlying cause: see below.

Underlying causes

A dog normally has a certain amount of 'friendly' bacteria on its skin which fight off infection. Occasionally, the friendly bacteria multiply to the extent that they begin to harm the dog, causing a number of diseases including:

Acute moist dermatitis: often referred to as 'wet eczema', this gives symptoms of inflamed, wet and painful sores. It is particularly common in long-haired dogs, and is probably the result of other conditions, such as parasite infestations (see pp. 66–71) or anal sac disorder (see p. 38).

Callus pyoderma: affecting larger dogs, this is the infection of the thick skin that covers the dog's bony protuberances, such as his elbows.

Impetigo: an infection that occurs in young dogs between about three and 12 months old, often referred to as 'puppy pyoderma'. The condition manifests itself with small, pus-filled spots on the puppy's abdomen, which rupture and leave yellow scabs.

Inter-digital pyoderma: as the name suggests, this condition affects the skin

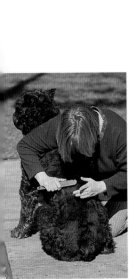

Regular grooming of your dog will help reveal any skin problems before they become serious.

⊙ COST

There are many different underlying causes of pyoderma, so the actual cause, and therefore the treatment, may be difficult to discover. The vet will need to charge you for his time and the drugs that he has used.

URGENCY INDICATOR

Pyoderma can cause discomfort to the affected dog, and may leave scarring, once the condition has been cleared up. Any dog affected by pyoderma should be taken for veterinary treatment as soon as the problem is first noticed.

DIAGNOSING PYODERM

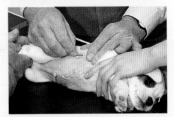

It is usual for a vet to take skin scrapes to establish the bacteria that is causing the pyoderma. ⊚

between the dog's toes or digits, and is often triggered by the presence of a foreign body, such as a piece of salt grit or grass seed. Matted fur between the toes may also trigger this condition, as may irritant chemicals (very often the disinfectant or detergent used to clean the dog's kennels). Where a dog is suffering from anal sac disorder (see p. 38) and is nibbling his feet, this can also cause inter-digital pyoderma.

Skin-fold pyoderma: folds of skin are inherently warm and damp, and this provides ideal conditions for the growth of bacteria. Obviously, breeds with large folds of skin, such as the sharpei, are more susceptible to this condition, although it also affects overweight bitches of any breed, affecting the folds of skin around the vulva.

Owner action

Ensure your dog is groomed on a regular basis; this will reveal pyoderma before it becomes severe.

Treatment

Antibiotics are used to treat all types of pyoderma. They may be in the form of shampoos, topical ointments or creams, or antibiotic medicines. The whole course of any antibiotics should be completed.

Seborrhoea

An abnormal/excessive secretion from the dog's sebaceous glands. Under normal circumstances, the skin renews cells at the same rate that cells die. When this balance becomes affected, new cells are not produced at the same rate as the old cells die off and the thickness of the skin is affected.

Symptoms

Areas of dead skin will become visible. These areas will appear flaky or greasy and may exhibit signs of inflammation.

Underlying causes

The causes may include pyoderma (see p. 72), ectoparasite infestations (see pp. 66–71), hot, dry conditions, use of incorrect shampoos and/or grooming techniques, nutritional disorders, hypothyroidism, Cushing's disease (see p. 99), or maybe diabetes mellitus (see p. 28). It is also believed that some forms of seborrhoea are hereditary in breeds, such as the Basset hound.

Owner action

Regular grooming together with parasite control, a good diet and control of the dog's environment (avoiding dry, hot surroundings) will all help prevent this condition occurring.

Treatment

Depending on the cause of the problem, treatment for seborrhoea may include antibiotics, especially if the condition has led to the dog developing pyoderma, and anti-inflammatory drug therapy in cases where the dog's skin is extremely inflamed and sore. Often, simply adding fat (vegetable or animal) to a dog's diet will help a mild case of seborrhoea. If the condition is caused by a flea infestation, a

DIAGNOSING SEBORRHOEA

Skin scrapes, blood tests and laboratory analysis of skin and hair samples will help the vet to diagnose and treat the problem.

course of anti-parasite powders, sprays or 'spot-ons' (drugs that are literally spotted on to the affected area) will be needed.

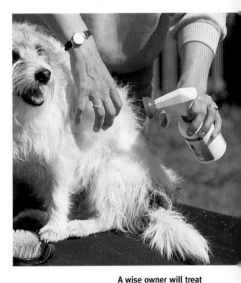

A wise owner will treat their dog with anti-parasitic sprays on a regular basis, rather than wait for a problem to occur.

COST

None of the treatments for seborrhoea is expensive, nor do they involve a lot of veterinary time, so the cost of treatment will be low.

Male dog problems

There are certain conditions and problems that only or mainly affect maledogs, in particular their reproductive system.

The normal male dog has two testes or testicles, which are contained in the scrotum, a pouch of skin that hangs between the dog's rear legs; it is in these testes that spermatozoa are produced. The spermatozoa are passed down to the epididymis, where they are stored. When the dog is mating, the spermatozoa pass through tubes to the urethra (the tube that carries urine away from the bladder), where they are mixed with fluid from the prostate and other glands.

The mixture formed is known as semen, and is ejaculated through the dog's penis during mating. Testosterone, the male sex hormone, is also produced by the testes, and it is this hormone which produces the secondary male characteristics. These characteristics include the heavy musculature of the male dog, and the erectile tissue in his penis. Normally, a dog's testes descend into his scrotum at about ten days old.

The sexual behaviour of male dogs

- The dog will reach sexual activity at between six and 12 months, although some sexual behaviour may be seen in male puppies as young as six or seven weeks.
- Although a dog may be sexually mature at one year of age, it is inadvisable to use him for stud (breeding) purposes until he is about 15 months old, and you have had the opportunity to evaluate his qualities fully.
- In breeds where there are some hereditary conditions or diseases, ensure that your dog has been examined by a vet.
- Male dogs are sexually active throughout the year, but are more likely to be sexually active in the summer months.

Although the age at which male dogs will cease to be fertile varies from breed to breed, seminal fluid quality will deteriorate from about seven years of age.

Aggression

There are many different types of aggression, each of which will require different treatments.

Symptoms
Change of mood, unpredictability of your dog's behaviour, aggressive behaviour.

Underlying causes
The different types of aggression are as follows:
- fear induced
- pain induced
- dominance
- territorial
- play
- competitive
- pathophysiological
- possessive
- predatory

These types of aggression, with the exception of pathophysiological aggression, are all behavioural in nature. Pathophysiological aggression is due to medical disorders.

Owner action
Take note of what your dog does, and of exactly what seems to trigger his aggressive behaviour.

Treatment
In the past, a vet presented with an aggressive male dog would probably have recommended that the dog was castrated (neutered), by surgical removal of his testicles. This operation was seen as a cure for all types of aggression in male dogs. Today, as more vets and lay people are becoming more educated on such matters, this is no longer the case, although there may be some advantages in having a dog castrated. This procedure may change the dog's nature. Where a

dog is castrated before reaching puberty, the dog may fail to develop his secondary sexual characteristics. It is also possible that such action will result in a change to the dog's metabolic rate, causing him to experience problems with weight control. However, where a dog is castrated after puberty, provided that proper dietary controls are exercised, there should be no major problems associated with the neutering.

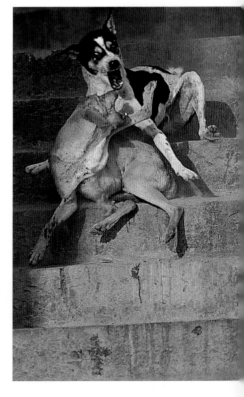

A dog which suddenly becomes extremely aggressive towards other dogs is showing the type of aggression which may need to be tackled by your vet.

Sexual Behaviour

Anorchia and cryptorchidism

Some dogs can and do become a nuisance at times, with what is known as 'anti-social' behaviour. Thankfully, this behaviour is usually only short term in most cases.

Where a dog's testes are both absent as a result of a natural phenomenon, the condition is known as anorchia. This is very rare. Chryptorchidism is when the testicles have not descended.

Symptoms
The dog will frequently mount other animals, small children, and even the legs of human adults.

Symptoms
In normal male dogs, both testes can be seen when the dog is a few weeks old. If this is not the case, then there could be a potentially serious problem, particularly if you intend to breed from or show the dog. Monorchids have one testicle that has descended, with the other hidden, while cryptorchids have no testicles descended. The term cryptorchid literally translates to 'hidden testicle'. The lack of one or both testes must be investigated. If a dog has had both testes removed surgically, he is referred to as a castrate.

Underlying causes
Such behaviour is linked to the androgens, the male sex hormones. However, most 'entire' (not neutered) male dogs never cause any problems.

Owner action
Try to be understanding towards the dog, and never physically punish him for his actions. Long walks and plenty of vigorous exercise may help reduce the frequency of the behaviour.

Treatment
If a dog's owner does not wish to have the dog castrated, or in cases where the dog will be used for breeding purposes at some time in its life, chemical control of the dog's sexual urges is possible. This is brought about by the administration, by a vet, of hormones that will suppress the normal release of testosterone (a male sex hormone). The most common drugs used are known as progestogens, which act like female hormones, and reduce the dog's libido (sex drive) without affecting his fertility. These drugs may be given as a 'depot injection', where the effects of the injected drug last for some time, or as tablets on a daily basis.

Underlying causes
The causes of cryptorchidism could include the testicles being hidden in the abdomen, or in the passage through the various layers of the abdominal muscles. They may even be outside the muscles, but under the skin; if this is the case, they can be easily located by feeling carefully around the area.

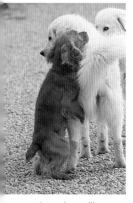

Some dogs will frequently try to mount other dogs, children and the legs of adults.

Testicular tumour

One of the most common cancers affecting dogs.

Symptoms

Alopecia (see p. 65), enlarged testicle(s), attractiveness to other male dogs.

Underlying causes

A study of confirmed testicular tumours diagnosed in over 400 dogs revealed that some breeds were at a higher risk than others. It was also found that cryptorchids (see p. 76) had a significantly higher risk than other intact dogs of contracting testicular cancer. Mechanisms that bring on testicular cancer may be both hereditary and environmental.

Owner action

Never adopt a 'wait and see' attitude to any unexplained lump or bump found on your dog. Delay can often mean the difference between successful treatment and the suffering or even death of the dog.

Treatment

Castration followed by drugs is the routine treatment, and this is usually beneficial. The drugs used are designed to kill any remaining cancer cells: this is known as chemotherapy.

DIAGNOSING TESTICULAR CANCER

The vet will carry out a physical examination, and ask details of the dog's clinical history. This will give the vet clues to the underlying cause of any lumps etc. Once a tumour is diagnosed, the vet may take biopsies from the affected testicle(s) to determine the extent of the condition.

DIAGNOSING TESTICULAR PROBLEMS

Usually, a physical examination will reveal the problem, although in some cases it will be necessary for the vet to use radiography or X-ray examination to show whether both testicles are present and exactly where they are located.

Owner action

Always check (or ask the vet to check) that both testicles are present and normal in any dog which you own or are considering buying.

Treatment

Almost every cryptorchid has problems as he would be severely penalized or even disqualified in the show ring (depending on the rules pertaining) and is almost invariably sterile (or at the very least has an extremely low sperm count). It is strongly recommended that, unless your dog is destined only to be a pet, or you had already decided to have him castrated, such animals should be avoided. Those who purchase such animals are strongly advised to have them surgically castrated at an early age.

COST

Could be high if there are any complications to the condition that require specialized or complicated surgery.

URGENCY INDICATOR

Any dog showing any of the symptoms of testicular cancer should be taken for veterinary examination as soon as possible. Any delay allows the condition to advance and makes it more difficult to treat.

COST

Treatment of most tumours can be prolonged and complicated, involving both surgery and drug therapy. As a consequence, the costs can be quite high.

Anal adenoma

Tumours around the anus, just under the skin. The adenoma is benign, that is not malignant (not fatal if left untreated), and there is a good chance of the dog making a complete recovery.

Symptoms

The tumours feel 'knobbly' to the touch. It is commonsense always to wash your hands and take other hygiene precautions if you are touching the dog in this area.

Underlying causes

Anal adenomas are directly linked to the androgens (male sex hormones) in older dogs, and this is quite a common problem.

DIAGNOSING ANAL ADENOMAS

Physical examination, sometimes coupled with radiography.

Owner action

Do not try to treat this condition as you might another area of infected skin. Seek veterinary advice and treatment as the condition is highly unlikely to heal itself.

Treatment

Anal adenomas can become very large and ulcerate, and the vet may decide to operate to improve the condition. As the tumour's growth depends upon the level of testosterone in the dog's body, the vet may recommend treatment with hormones that will suppress the normal release of testosterone. In some cases, surgical castration of the dog may be called for, and this will prevent the condition from recurring.

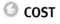

HOMEOPATHIC TREATMENT:
Thuja occidentalis is a wart remedy that may be effective for this condition. Ask the vet for advice.

COST
Relatively low, although costs will increase if surgery is necessary.

Prostate problems

Problems with the prostate gland, a gland that produces secretions which combine with spermatozoa and secretions from other glands to form semen. The prostate gland is at the base of the male dog's bladder, where the urethra (the tube that carries urine away from the bladder) begins. The gland itself surrounds the urethra. Because of its position, problems with the prostate gland can cause the dog to have great trouble urinating and even defecating.

DIAGNOSING PROSTATE PROBLEMS

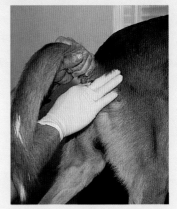

Diagnosis of the problem will consist of a physical examination of the dog's abdomen. In some cases, a catheter (a plastic tube) may be passed up the penis and blood and/or pus samples obtained; these will be sent for laboratory analysis. X-rays and ultrasound examinations may also be made by the vet, and in some cases a biopsy of the prostate gland may be necessary. A piece of the affected tissue is surgically removed, and then examined under a microscope in a veterinary laboratory.

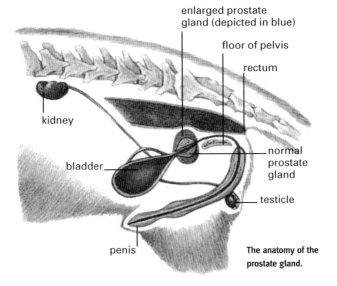

enlarged prostate
gland (depicted in blue)

floor of pelvis

rectum

kidney

normal
prostate
gland

bladder

testicle

penis

The anatomy of the
prostate gland.

Symptoms

May include constipation, incontinence, blood in the urine, a bleeding penis, pus from the penis, straining to pass feces and/or the production of ribbon-like feces.

Underlying causes

Sometimes, when a male dog is between six and ten years of age, the prostate begins to enlarge. This condition is known as hyperplasia, is painless, and is considered as quite normal by many vets. Another cause of prostate problems is when harmful bacteria get into the prostate gland and cause an infection; this is known as prostatitis.

Owner action

If the vet prescribes a course of antibiotics for your dog, ensure that the whole course is given regularly. It is also highly likely that the vet will want to see your dog frequently to check on the effectiveness of the treatment and the course of the dog's progress.

Treatment

Treatment depends upon the nature of the condition, but where the problem is hyperplasia, drug and/or hormone treatment may be given. In severe cases the vet may recommend that the affected dog is castrated.

In cases of prostatitis, long-term courses of antibiotics may be used.

 HOMEOPATHIC TREATMENT: Agnus castus, conium and selenium may be effective for this condition. The vet will advise you.

COST Depends on the severity of the problem, but costs are usually quite moderate.

Bitch problems

Like most other animals, dogs only mate when they are 'in season' or 'on heat'. Bitches only have one oestrus during each breeding season, during which they will accept a mating from a dog. As far as we know, this is unique in the animal kingdom, and it means that there are only a few days during each breeding season when the bitch can conceive. Vets can help determine the best days on which to have the bitch mated, namely those days when she is most likely to conceive; this is done either by taking vaginal smears, or by taking a blood sample and measuring the hormone levels. The vet is able to inform the breeder when the bitch is about to ovulate, that is when the eggs are about to be released from her ovaries, or when ovulation has just occurred. The breeder can then take the bitch to the stud dog during the bitch's peak of fertility.

Most bitches reach puberty at about six to seven months, but some may achieve puberty as early as four months, while others may not experience their first season until they are almost two years old. If a bitch has not had a season by the time she is two years old, then veterinary advice must be sought.

The bitch's reproductive system

A bitch has two ovaries, which produce the eggs, and these are fertilized in the Fallopian tubes, which lead to the uterus. The uterus is Y-shaped, and consists of two long horns. The fertilized eggs are carried to the horns of the uterus, where they are implanted. The foetuses grow in the horns of the uterus throughout the bitch's gestation period or pregnancy. The wall of the uterus consists of layers of smooth muscle, called the myometrium. At the base of the uterus is the cervix, a muscular organ which closes the uterus except when the bitch is mating or giving birth. The cervix is joined to the outside world by the vagina, and the vagina terminates as the vulva, or vaginal lips. Just inside the vagina is the 'vestibule', a chamber with extremely strong muscles in its wall. It is these muscles that help 'tie' the dog and bitch during mating.

If you do not intend to breed from a bitch, there are many advantages to having her spayed (neutered or sterilized) when she is young, as she will not then suffer from diseases of the ovaries or uterus, since they are removed in the operation. Obviously also you do not run the risk of unwanted pregnancies. In older 'entire' (unspayed) bitches, it is common to see pyometra (see p. 82), a life-threatening condition affecting the uterus. Entire bitches may also suffer pseudo or phantom pregnancies (see p. 81), and these can cause both physical and mental problems for the affected bitch.

Pseudo pregnancy

False or phantom pregnancy. A pseudo pregnancy may occur in a bitch that has failed to conceive in a given oestrus, and has different effects on different bitches.

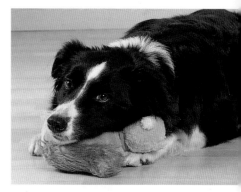

Symptoms

In some cases of pseudo pregnancy, the owner may not notice any difference in either the bitch's physical or mental condition. In other bitches, the pseudo pregnancy may mean that the dog's abdomen swells, her mammary glands (teats) fill with milk, and her mental attitude will change. She will spend much time nest-building, she will cry and be reluctant to take any exercise, and may even go through the pushing and thrusting of an actual birth. Many such bitches will form emotional attachments to inanimate objects, particularly their toys, and some have 'invisible' puppies. The bitch's territorial and maternal aggression will show, as she protects her invisible litter, and this can be extremely upsetting for the owner of the bitch. Many of the bitches that exhibit symptoms of pseudo pregnancy will show more marked symptoms season after season throughout their life.

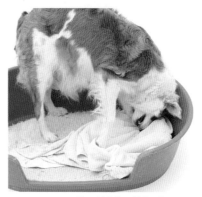

Top: **A bitch suffering from a pseudo pregnancy will often form strong emotional attachments to inanimate objects such as her toys.**
Above: **Nesting behaviour such as this in an unmated bitch is almost certainly a sign of a phantom pregnancy.**

Underlying causes

Pseudo pregnancies are triggered by the bitch's hormone levels. They are perfectly natural, and are nature's way of ensuring that, in a pack of wolves (the ancient ancestor of the domestic dog), there are many bitches producing milk, and capable of rearing or helping to rear a litter.

Owner action

It is always helpful in cases of pseudo pregnancy if the bitch is given more exercise than normal, and she is not allowed toys and similar objects to play with.

DIAGNOSING PSEUDO PREGNANCY

The vet will examine the bitch, to ensure that she is not actually pregnant.

Treatment

In severe cases, the vet may recommend that the bitch is given hormone treatment, although in mild cases, most vets will recommend that the bitch is left to go through the phase on her own.

Pyometra

Infection of the bitch's uterus.

Symptoms

The most obvious and earliest symptom of pyometra is an increased thirst, leading to increased drinking, leading in turn to increased urination. Other symptoms may include:

- a poor quality coat;
- reluctance to eat or even anorexia;
- vomiting;
- lethargy and a general reluctance to take any exercise;
- a discharge of mucus from the vulva after the season has finished;
- excessive licking of the vulva.

The infection causes the uterus to swell and fill with pus, and in some cases, the uterus can reach almost gigantic proportions. Once the condition is there, it will get progressively worse with every season that the bitch has.

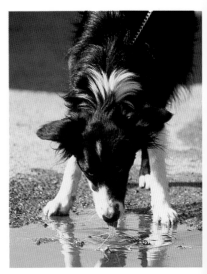

Increased thirst is the first and most obvious sign that your dog may be suffering form pyometra.

URGENCY INDICATOR

A severe case of pyometra can be life-threatening, so you should watch out for any of the symptoms listed above, which may appear within a few weeks of the bitch's oestrus. If your bitch is exhibiting any of these symptoms, you should seek veterinary advice as soon as possible.

🔋 COST

Surgery will be involved, and in severe cases intensive care will be needed. The costs could be quite high.

Underlying causes

Pyometra is caused by bacteria, probably from the bitch's urinary system, and it is believed that the higher than normal hormone levels present in the bitch during oestrus may help promote the growth of the bacteria. Spayed bitches cannot develop pyometra.

DIAGNOSING PYOMETRA

As this is a common problem with bitches, the vet will easily recognize the signs of pyometra, and act accordingly. Occasionally, a vet may use X-ray and ultrasound examinations to confirm his diagnosis, or he may take samples of any discharge from the vulva; these will be sent for laboratory analysis.

Owner action

There is little that the owner of an affected bitch can do other than seek advice from the vet.

Treatment

The treatment for pyometra is for the bitch to be spayed as soon as possible, unless she is too ill for the operation. If this is the case, the vet will treat the bitch with antibiotics and maybe an intravenous drip, until she is well enough for the operation.

Mammary cancer

Cancer of the breast. Extremely common in unspayed bitches, almost half of all mammary tumours are malignant (progressively worsening and invariably fatal if left untreated). As veterinary science advances, more and more is discovered about tumours, and how to treat them successfully.

Symptoms
Lumps in the bitch's mammary glands ('teats').

Underlying causes
Not entirely known, but the condition is believed to be linked with hormones in many cases.

Owner action
There is little that the owner of an affected bitch can do other than seek advice from the vet.

Treatment
The treatment for mammary tumours may include surgery (cutting out or reducing the tumour), chemotherapy (the use of drugs to kill or shrink the tumour), radiotherapy (radiation given to destroy diseased tissue, often used in conjunction with surgery), or hyperthermia. The latter involves the application of extremely high temperatures to a tumour, via ultrasound or electromagnetic radiation.

Many tumours that at one stage were felt to be beyond treatment are now being successfully treated, leading to an improvement in a dog's quality of life, and a longer life.

DIAGNOSING MAMMARY CANCER

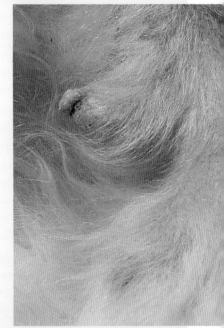

A typical mammary tumour will appear as a well-defined lump in the bitch's teat. It may only be the size of a pea when first noticed, but the lump will increase in size as the bitch comes into oestrus.

To identify whether the problem is a tumour, the vet may use many types of examination, including physical, X-ray, ultrasound and blood tests. Once a tumour is confirmed, further tests will be necessary before treatment can begin. These tests will be to identify the tumour's type, size, exact location and the degree to which it may have spread. As this is such a specialized area, the vet may refer you to a specialist vet.

Mastitis

The inflammation of the bitch's mammary glands during lactation (the production of milk to feed a litter).

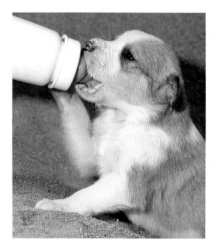

Where a bitch is suffering from acute mastitis, it will be necessary to hand rear the pups.

Symptoms

Mastitis results in hard teats that feel hot to the touch; any milk produced by an infected teat may be bloodstained and/or look abnormal. The affected bitch will be 'off colour'; she will almost certainly have little or no appetite, and may vomit.

Underlying causes

Mastitis is caused by bacterial infection by streptococci bacteria.

DIAGNOSING MASTITIS

Mastitis can be diagnosed by physical examination by a vet.

Owner action

While any teat is not functioning properly, it will be necessary to check the litter even more carefully than usual to ensure that they are getting enough milk. If there are several teats affected by mastitis, and so not delivering enough – or even any – milk, it may be necessary to hand rear one or more puppies.

To help prevent mastitis, wipe the bitch's abdomen clean on a regular basis, preferably using a mild anti-bacterial cleaner which the vet will recommend. The pups should also be encouraged to use all teats evenly, although this may not be possible where the litter is very small. In such cases, careful hand stripping of the milk in the unused teats may be called for. The vet will demonstrate how to do this. Throughout hand stripping, ensure that you maintain the highest degree of personal hygiene, and wash your hands before and after the procedure; it is also advisable to wash your hands between teats to avoid transferring the infection.

Treatment

Antibiotics will be necessary for the successful treatment of mastitis, so veterinary advice should be sought as soon as possible. Often, carefully stripping of the milk by hand will be necessary (see above), and the bitch will get some relief from having the affected mammary gland(s) bathed in warm water. In very rare cases, lancing or surgery may be necessary. Where proper treatment is sought and given, most cases of mastitis will clear up within 36–48 hours.

RELATED CONDITIONS WHICH MAY PRODUCE SIMILAR SYMPTOMS

A bitch suffering a pseudo pregnancy (see p. 81) may also develop mastitis.

Eclampsia

'Milk fever' or lactation tetany, which is the paralysis of milk production in the dam's teats.

Symptoms

An affected bitch will be anxious and will shy away from light. She may totally ignore her puppies, often wandering away from them, salivate profusely and be extremely uncoordinated. The bitch's body temperature will rise from 39°C to 41°C (102°F to 106°F) or even higher, her heart rate will increase, and she will have convulsions.

Underlying causes

Lower than normal levels of calcium and possibly glucose in the bitch's blood may trigger this condition, although the actual cause is unknown. Eclampsia in bitches is seen after whelping. The smaller breeds are more susceptible to the condition, which can occur up to 21 days after whelping, although – very rarely – it can occur just prior to whelping.

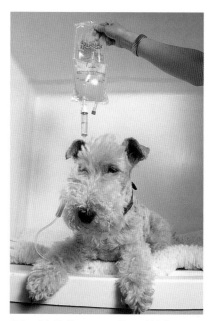

Above: **A bitch suffering from eclampsia may need calcium and glucose via an intravenous drip.**

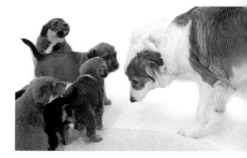

Below: **It is highly unlikely that eclampsia will affect this bitch now, as her pups are too old.**

DIAGNOSING ECLAMPSIA

Physical examination.

URGENCY INDICATOR

Contact the vet immediately. If the convulsions are not treated, the dog will die. Eclampsia is an emergency.

Owner action

As this is such an extremely serious condition, veterinary treatment must be sought immediately, and there is nothing that the owner can do. **Under no circumstances should anyone try to hold down a fitting dog.** This can cause further damage to the bitch, and may injure the person attempting to hold her down.

Treatment

The vet will treat the condition with cal-cium and glucose, which may be delivered via intraperitoneal injections (injections into the abdomen) or an intravenous drip. The results of this treatment really are spectacular, as the affected bitch can recover in just a few minutes.

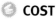

COST

Injections are low cost; if intravenous drips are required these will be more expensive.

Nymphomania

Bitches with increased sexual drive or unusual oestrus cycles.

Symptoms

While this term may be given to bitches who have increased sexual drive (libido), it is also used to describe bitches who have more oestruses than normal, where pro-oestrus (the beginning stage of oestrus) is abnormally long, and those bitches which show more than normal interest in male dogs.

DIAGNOSING NYMPHOMANIA

Other than observing the symptoms already described, there is no method of diagnosing this condition.

Underlying causes

It is thought that the condition is caused by enlarged ovarian follicles (cavities in the ovary) producing too much oestrogen (a female sex hormone).

Owner action

When on heat, bitches will often mount other bitches, and the owner should not prevent this if the bitches concerned are to be used for breeding purposes.

Treatment

In chronic cases where the bitch will not be used for breeding purposes, spaying is the best treatment. In other cases, hormone injections will probably work.

Metritis

Infection of the inner lining of the uterus, the endometrium.

Symptoms

Include a foul-smelling discharge from the bitch's vulva, lack of appetite, reduced milk production, and vomiting.

DIAGNOSING METRITIS

Physical examination, which is often supported by laboratory analysis of the discharge.

Underlying causes

The condition is caused by a bacterial infection, and occurs just after whelping.

Owner action

Try to keep the bitch clean during whelping, and ensure that the area in and around her whelping box is clean. If it is necessary to assist the bitch manually during whelping, then it is almost certain that she will require antibiotics administered by a vet in order to prevent the onset of metritis.

Treatment

Treatment will consist of antibiotics, and the bitch may be given supportive drugs to help her fight the condition such as prostaglandin, which will help to open the cervix and expel the infective contents.

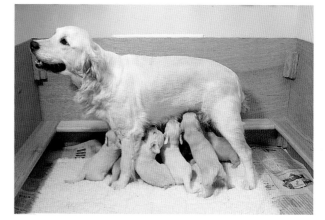

Vaginal prolapse will usually occur after whelping. Today whelping boxes are not always popular with vets.

Vaginal prolapse or hyperplasia

When the lining of the vagina prolapses through the vulva.

Symptoms

In older, entire bitches, who have had many oestrus cycles, the lining of the vagina may be seen as a red, swollen mass protruding from the vulva. In some cases, the mass may be as big as a large chicken's egg.

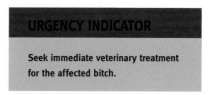

URGENCY INDICATOR

Seek immediate veterinary treatment for the affected bitch.

Underlying causes

Usually occurs after whelping. It is caused by the reaction of the lining of the vagina (the vaginal mucosa) to the hormone oestrogen. This results in the vaginal mucosa developing excessive folding, and these folds may protrude through the bitch's vulva. The condition is particularly common in boxers and bulldogs.

DIAGNOSING HYPERPLASIA

Physical examination by a vet.

Owner action

Keep the protruding folds of mucosa clean, avoiding any contamination with feces, urine etc., while veterinary treatment is sought.

Treatment

Antibiotics will be needed to prevent infection. In mild cases, it is necessary only to keep the mucosa clean, as the folds will regress spontaneously during the period of the bitch's season when she is not in oestrus. Surgery is often necessary in chronic cases, and where the condition recurs regularly, spaying is the best course of action.

☀ COST

The administration of antibiotics to ward off infections will not be expensive, but the costs will increase if surgery is necessary.

Vaginitis

Infection of the vagina leading to inflammation.

Symptoms
Typically, a thick, creamy discharge will be seen from the lips of the vulva, and the bitch will probably spend much time licking her vulva in an attempt to remove this discharge.

Underlying causes
Vaginitis is caused by harmful bacteria. There are many different bacteria that can cause this condition, and these must be positively and expertly identified before any treatment can be given.

Owner action
If you have more than one bitch, such as in breeding kennels, it is a wise precaution to isolate the affected bitch to prevent the spread of the infection, and to have all cases of vaginitis treated as soon as possible.

Treatment
A course of antibiotics. These should be taken as directed, and the course must be completed.

DIAGNOSING VAGINITIS

Vaginal swabs are taken by the vet pushing a large 'cotton bud' inside the bitch's vulva, where it is used to take a smear from the mucus lining the vagina. This sample is cultured in a laboratory and the bacteria responsible for the infection are identified. Many laboratories also carry out tests to find the most effective antibiotic for the specific infection.

Misalliance

A mating that was not intended.

Owner action
To prevent misalliance occurring, take care to ensure that your bitch is not let out of your sight when she is in season.

Treatment
The vet will administer an injection of hormones. These injections override the effects of the bitch's own hormones, making her body believe that she is not pregnant, and causing oestrus to begin again. Vets do not like to give such injections as a matter of course, since they can sometimes have very serious side effects, including the development of pyometra (see p. 82). Prevention is always better than cure, and so all bitches in season, and therefore receptive to the attentions of a male dog, must be very carefully monitored and kept well out of trouble or temptation.

URGENCY INDICATOR

When a bitch has mated accidentally, and you do not want her to have the litter, it is vital that you contact the vet within 48 hours of the misalliance.

COST
All that is required is an injection, so costs will be relatively low.

URGENCY INDICATOR

Seek veterinary treatment within 24 hours otherwise the condition will become acute and will be more difficult to treat.

COST
Modern antibiotics are effective and cost relatively little.

Toxocara canis

An internal parasite that infects pregnant or nursing bitches, and also young puppies.

Symptoms

Toxocara canis is a white worm, measuring between 8 cm and 15 cm (3¼ and 6 in) long, and pointed at both ends. Although often passed with feces, sometimes these worms will appear as a white coiled spring out of the anus. In a very few though well-publicized cases children have become infected with Toxocara canis, causing blindness.

Underlying causes

Normally, larvae will lie dormant in a bitch, but they are activated by the release of the hormones associated with pregnancy. The resulting worms will migrate around the bitch's body, including across the placenta and into the litter. The bitch's litter will be born with larvae already in their bodies, and will acquire more from the bitch's milk and saliva as she carries out her maternal duties, such as cleaning and feeding the puppies. In addition, the bitch will be infected with even more worms as she licks the puppies and cleans up their feces. The feces from infected bitches and puppies will pass the eggs of *Toxocara canis* into the environment, where they can lie dormant for many months before finding their way into a new host, and continuing the cycle.

Owner action

In young puppies, a heavy infestation may be life-threatening. In order to minimize the problems that an infestation of *Toxocara canis* can cause, it is vital that all bitches are wormed before mating, during their pregnancy and throughout lactation. Puppies should be wormed at two-week intervals between the ages of

DIAGNOSING *TOXOCARA*

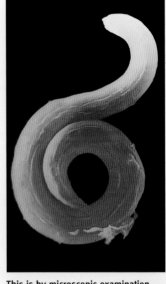

This is by microscopic examination of fecal matter.

three and 12 weeks. After that, they should be wormed at least every 12 weeks until they are 12 months of age, and then at least every six months.

Take commonsense hygiene precautions such as washing your hands after touching your dog, and always before eating, to ensure your own health is not affected by this dangerous parasite.

Treatment

Oral administration of wormers in the form of tablets, liquids or pastes.

WARNING: REMEMBER THAT *TOXOCARA CANIS* IS ZOONOTIC.

Problems suffered by elderly dogs

Old age brings with it certain conditions, mainly caused by the effects of wear and tear on the body and its organs. As veterinary science advances, coupled with similar advances in the production of dog foods, dogs are living longer and healthier lives. The average life span of breeds of dog varies tremendously with, in general, smaller breeds living longer than the giant breeds. The giant breeds may only have a life span of seven or eight years, while smaller breeds can live well into their teens, with the average life span for a dog being about 12 years. Good husbandry, including good nutrition, checking a puppies' parents for hereditary diseases, and good medical care, can all increase both the quality and length of a dog's life.

Symptoms and needs of elderly dogs

- An elderly dog will require more rest than when it was younger, and will sleep very deeply.
- Hair will grey in many dogs, although this greying may start well before the stage where the dog could be described as elderly.
- He may not wish to exercise anywhere near as much as he used to, and his appetite may change.
- Elderly dogs should not be subjected to extremes of temperature, so do not put your dog out on a cold night.
- Do not let him sleep on a cold concrete floor. Concrete is notoriously cold and damp, and will exacerbate any conditions from which he is already suffering, such as arthritis. A bean bag is an ideal bed for an elderly dog, as it will insulate the dog and make him very comfortable.
- Mineral supplements may be necessary. Always consult the vet before you give any supplement to your dog.

Many problems and medical conditions which, while the dog was young, were considered minor and of little consequence, may become more serious as the dog ages. The following are some of the problems and conditions which are particularly common in older dogs.

ANAL SAC DISEASE   38
An uncomfortable condition which shouldbe relieved as soon as possible.
ARTHRITIS   42
All cases of osteoarthritis should be treated seriously.
BLINDNESS   21
Refer all eye conditions and injuries to a vet immediately.
BRONCHITIS   54
Never ignore any symptoms of a possible bronchial infection, even if mild. Seek veterinary advice.
COAT PROBLEMS   92
This condition should be treated, as it will irritate your dog, leading to further deterioration.
CONSTIPATION   35
Refer all cases of constipation to a vet.
DEAFNESS   10
Seek veterinary advice sooner rather than later.
HEART DISEASE   59 & 62
See a vet immediately if you suspect your dog has a heart problem.
INCONTINENCE   93
Seek veterinary advice as incontinence can be a symptom of several other serious diseases.
KIDNEY FAILURE   36
Contact your vet straight away if you suspect your dog has kidney failure, as it is life-threatening.
LIVER FAILURE   94
Be on the lookout for any indication that the dog is 'off-colour' and if so, seek veterinary treatment.
LOSS OF APPETITE   23–27
If you suspect that the loss of appetite is due to a blockage of the digestive system, seek veterinary advice immediately.
OBESITY   95
Obesity is a major cause of many potentially life-threatening diseases, so get advice as soon as possible.
SENILITY   91
Take your dog to the vet for examination, as it may be possible to administer drugs that will help him.
TOOTH DECAY   94
Seek advice as it may be possible to improve your dog's quality of life.

Senility

The mental deterioration of an animal due (usually) to old age.

Symptoms
As your dog reaches old age, you will notice that on some days in particular he may be more restless and disorientated, while on other days, he will seem to behave perfectly normally. Often, a dog suffering from senility will seem to want to spend more time in the company of his owner, and demand more attention from members of the human family.

DIAGNOSING SENILITY
It is extremely difficult to diagnose senility accurately, other than to take account of the dog's symptoms, age etc.

Underlying causes
Senility is almost always due to the normal ageing process, whereby damaged cells, in this case in the brain, are no longer being replaced. In some cases, diseases can affect the brain and damage the cells, causing senility.

Owner action
In most cases, what is needed is plenty of tender loving care and more than a little understanding by members of the dog's human family.

Treatment
There is no cure for senility. Any drug therapy used by the vet will be to improve your dog's quality of life.

URGENCY INDICATOR
If your dog shows these symptoms, you should take him to the vet for examination, as it may be possible to administer drugs that will help him.

COST
Due to a lack of real treatment, the only costs involved are those of drug therapy and veterinary consultation, and these are likely to be low.

Coat problems

As in all mammals, a dog's coat will be affected by the passing of time. This may involve changes in texture and/or thinning of the hair. Many of the 'problems' associated with the dog's coat are simply part of the ageing process and therefore inevitable. However, it is still possible in many cases to alleviate the problems.

Symptoms

The dog's coat may become greasier or drier, and tends to become matted and 'tatty' very easily. At the same time, the nails may begin to grow faster (or seem to wear down at a slower rate).

Regular bathing and grooming of your dog's coat will help prevent many skin problems from occurring.

DIAGNOSING COAT PROBLEMS

There could be several reasons for your dog's condition, so the vet will need to carry out a physical examination and in some cases blood samples may also be tested. These tests will be looking for the underlying cause of the dog's poor coat, as it may be due to the ageing process or could be caused by skin disease or infestation by ectoparasites etc.

Underlying causes

As a dog gets older, the texture and character of his coat will change. These changes are due to hormone levels associated with the dog's ageing process. Nails grow longer due to both this and the inevitable decrease in exercise.

Owner action

To keep the coat in good condition, bath and groom your dog at more regular intervals, and also check his nails, clipping them as and when necessary. Before attempting to trim your dog's nails, you should seek the advice and guidance of the vet, as incorrect cutting can cause severe pain and discomfort for your dog. Where your dog's claws are light in colour, it is easy to see the 'quick' and avoid cutting into it, but in dogs with black claws this is far more difficult. The claw should be cut just in front of the 'quick', using clippers designed for the task. **Never use scissors to cut claws, as they can easily rip out the claw rather than actually cutting it.**

It may be advantageous with some dogs to have the coat clipped out; this will be extremely beneficial to breeds that have long coats liable to become matted, such as the Old English sheepdog.

Treatment

Treatment for coat conditions is usually based on diet. Dry coats will need more oil or fat in the diet, while greasy coats will need less. Seek veterinary advice and guidance before changing your dog's diet.

Incontinence

Incontinence may be urinary (see p. 37), fecal or both.

Symptoms

Your dog will have 'accidents' with his toileting, often extremely frequently. If your dog experiences only the occasional mishap, it is unlikely that he is actually incontinent.

Underlying causes

As the dog ages, muscles become inefficient, and this can lead to incontinence. Fecal incontinence may be caused by a flabby anal sphincter muscle (the ring of muscle that opens the anus to the outside).

Prostate gland problems (see p. 78) are one of the most common causes of urinary incontinence in the male dog, and cystitis (see p. 33) is the most common cause in bitches, although faulty or 'lazy' urethral valves may also be the cause. Urethral valves control the flow of urine, and are muscles situated around the urethra. In 'lazy' valves, the muscles do not seal off the urethra properly, or, in some cases, do not seal it off at all. Any such problem should be investigated by the vet.

In many cases, wet beds are simply the result of the dog feeling unable or unwilling to make the effort to get up. Arthritis (see p. 42) is a major cause of an elderly dog lacking the will to move.

Owner action

Serilize a small glass bottle that has a good seal, by boiling it in water for about ten minutes. When it has drained, use it to take a sample of the dog's urine, which the vet can then test to find the underlying causes of your dog's incontinence.

Treatment

If the problem is associated with an infection (for example, cystitis), a course of antibiotics will be necessary. In some cases, especially where the affected animal is a recently spayed bitch, hormone treatment will be necessary.

URGENCY INDICATOR

On its own, incontinence is not serious, but if the urine is tinged with blood, or your dog appears to be in pain when he passes urine, urgent veterinary advice should be sought, as incontinence can be a symptom of several other serious diseases such as cancer.

DIAGNOSING CAUSES OF INCONTINENCE

Very often, the problem is a symptom of other diseases, so your vet will carry out a thorough physical examination of your dog. In many cases, urine samples will be sent for laboratory analysis to find any underlying causes.

COST

Most costs involved in treating incontinence are low, although where there are complications, perhaps leading to surgery on the dog, costs will inevitably increase.

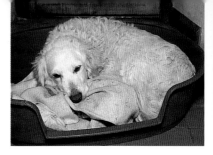

Liver failure

The liver is one of the main organs of the dog's body, and has many complex roles to perform. These roles include helping the kidneys remove waste products from the dog's body, the production of proteins involved in blood clotting, the processing and storing of fats and carbohydrates, production of bile (necessary for digestion), and the general purification of the blood. Any major problems with the liver will be serious.

A dog which is off-colour and spends more time than usual in his bed may be showing symptoms of liver failure.

Symptoms

Symptoms can be very difficult to detect, particularly in the early stages of this condition. They may include the dog going off his food, weight loss, vomiting, diarrhoea or general lack of condition in the dog. In addition, the white of the eye will turn yellow.

DIAGNOSING LIVER FAILURE

The vet will do blood and urine tests to look for any abnormalities, and may need to take X-rays and ultrasound examinations to see any physical changes.

Underlying causes

Long-term inflammation of the liver, cancer, or problems with the bile duct (the tube down which bile passes) can all be causes of liver failure.

Owner action

There is very little that an owner of a dog with diagnosed liver disease can do, apart from supplying tender loving care.

URGENCY INDICATOR

As symptoms of liver failure are vague, you should be on the lookout for any indication that the dog is 'off-colour' and, as in all such cases, seek veterinary treatment. It is a sad fact that many animals die due to their owners ignoring subtle changes in behaviour.

COST

Due to the difficulties in treatment, and the many possible underlying causes of liver disease, the costs of treatment for an affected dog are likely to be quite high.

Treatment

Unfortunately, there is often very little that can be done for a dog suffering from chronic liver failure. Any treatment given to an affected dog will be to help alleviate the symptoms, and give the dog a reasonable standard of life. In order to reduce the build-up of waste products which cause any liver problems, the vet may put your dog on a special low-protein diet. A reduction in the stress of the dog's life will also be beneficial, and allow him to obtain the rest he will need. In many cases, the vet will also instigate drug therapy, to reduce the build-up of fluids in the dog's abdomen, and antibiotics will be used to fight specific infections. If the quality of life drops, the owner must decide, taking advice and guidance from the vet, when it is necessary to end the dog's suffering. It is impossible to say how long a dog affected by liver disease will live an acceptable life; the vet will advise you on your individual case.

Tooth decay

If an elderly dog's teeth become diseased, he may show a reluctance to eat his food, particularly if the food is hard (such as biscuits). Examination of his teeth may reveal obvious 'bad' (decayed) teeth, or halitosis (bad breath – see p. 23). A veterinary examination will reveal whether any treatment can be given, which will improve the dog's quality of life.

Obesity

Many older dogs become overweight, and this can cause all sorts of problems.

Symptoms

Excess covering of flesh hiding the dog's ribs, which should normally be visible under the skin, particularly as the dog exercises. Other symptoms are waddling, sluggish movements, and difficulty and reluctance in exercising.

DIAGNOSING OBESITY

It is possible to obtain tables giving the ideal weight ranges for different breeds, but most vets will not adhere to them too firmly, as they are only a guide. Each dog is an individual, and needs to be treated as such. Common sense will guide you as to whether your dog has a weight problem, and the vet will advise you on how best to tackle the situation.

Underlying causes

As he gets older, and no longer wishes to take as much exercise as he once did, your dog may put on weight; this extra weight will make him more prone to many diseases, including heart problems. See 'Eating and Drinking' pp.22–39. Any breed of dog can become obese, and in many cases this is due to the owner's actions – giving the wrong diet, too many treats, not enough exercise – and therefore avoidable.

Owner action

If your dog is overweight, you will need to adjust his diet. This can be done in one of two ways. Firstly, you could reduce the amount of food that you feed him; how-

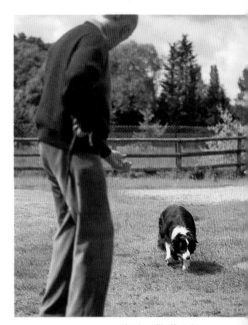

Obesity will affect the health and wellbeing of any dog, and prevent him from enjoying his exercise.

ever, many dogs then address their constant hunger by scavenging, even if they never did this in their earlier years. Secondly, and most agree that this is the best method, you could change his diet for one of the many low calorie diets specifically produced by food manufacturers for elderly dogs. These foods may also help prevent or alleviate some of the problems that may affect older dogs. Always consult the vet before drastically changing your dog's diet. Many vets have a trained dietary adviser.

If you feed a mix of meat (either tinned or fresh) and biscuit, the you should change the biscuits for a low-calorie type to reduce the total amount of calories that your dog ingests each day. The biscuits, in whole or in part, can also be substituted with cooked vegetables to help reduce the weight of your dog.

WARNING: OBESITY IS VERY DANGEROUS TO A DOG OF ANY AGE.

Other medical disorders

There are some problems that cannot easily be categorized, but that may still affect your dog. This chapter gives information on the main conditions.

Behaviour problems

Throughout a dog's life, his behaviour will change in small ways. When you notice any behavioural changes, you should make a note of them and, if the problem persists, veterinary advice should be sought. If any aspect of the dog's behaviour gives you cause for concern, do not hesitate to contact the vet for advice. Many problems are far easier to treat if caught early, rather than left until the problem has developed into a major, possibly life-threatening, condition.

Some common changes in behaviour are:

Loss of appetite: This may be due to mouth ulcers, congestion of the nose, an infectious disease or a metabolic disease (one that affects the body's ability to properly digest and utilize food).

Pica: A craving for unnatural foods, which may result from a poor diet. In such cases, affected dogs may eat their own droppings, the faeces of farm animals, such as cows or horses, or even stones, rocks and pebbles. Where a dog eats faecal matter, this is known as coprophagy.

Insatiable appetite: Especially when this is accompanied by weight loss, the dog may have a problem with his pancreas or be suffering from a large infestation of worms. The pancreas secretes enzymes to aid digestion, so any problems with the pancreas will affect the dog's appetite.

Polydipsia: Excessive thirst. This may be caused by something as simple as feeding a dry diet or a diet high in salts, or even by stress. It may also be caused by hot weather, and is perfectly normal in lactating bitches and even in bitches experiencing a pseudo pregnancy (see p. 81). However, it can also be indicative of more serious ailments, such as kidney problems (see p. 36) or liver disease (see p. 94), so must be investigated by a vet.

Pacing, panting, whining, barking, scratching at the floor or bedding: These are all signs of restlessness in a dog. They may indicate that the dog feels uncomfortable, or is in pain; that the room temperature is too hot or too cold; that he needs to go to the toilet; that he is lonely or that he is bored. If your dog has had dressings put on an injury or wound, these may be too tight, and this will also make the dog feel restless. Dependent upon the cause, steps should always be taken to alleviate a dog's distress if this is at all possible.

Physiological problems

Other changes that you may observe will be physiological. Some common physiological changes are:

Polyuria: Production of large amounts of urine. This may be as a direct result of polydipsia (see above), or could be due to problems with the kidneys (see p. 36), liver failure (see p. 94) or diabetes mellitus (see p. 28).

Constipation: (see p. 35).

Diarrhoea: (see p.32). To help the vet identify the cause of diarrhoea, which is a symptom of many different conditions, you should note the frequency, colour, smell and consistency of the motions passed by your dog.

Vomiting: (see p. 30). To help the vet correctly and speedily identify the cause of this symptom, the frequency and volume of vomit should be noted, as should the presence of blood or mucus in the vomit.

Vaginal discharge: This is often an indica-

tion of vaginitis (see p. 88) or pyoderma (see p. 72) and should always be investigated by a vet.

Nasal discharge: Discharge from the nose. This may be due to infection (for example, a cold), the presence of a foreign body, or the dog may be in the early stages of a viral disease.

Aural discharge: Discharge from the ears. This is a sign of ear diseases such as otitis (see p. 12).

Ocular discharge: Discharge from the eye(s). This is an indication of eye problems such as conjunctivitis (see p. 17).

Changes in the colour of the dog's mucus membranes: The best way to see this is to examine the inside of the dog's mouth, particularly his gums. Pale gums may indicate anaemia (see p. 63), haemorrhage or heart problems (see p.59 and 62). Gums that appear slightly blue (cyanosis) may indicate a breathing problem. Gums that appear to have a yellow tinge (jaundice) may indicate that the dog has liver problems (see p. 94), or the disease leptospirosis. Leptospirosis is often called 'rat-catcher's yellows' or 'Weil's disease'. It is zoonotic, so can be transmitted to humans, and is often fatal. In young puppies, leptospirosis may manifest itself in the sudden death of one or more of the pups in the litter, often without any prior indication of ill health. Symptoms vary but may include anorexia, lethargy, jaundice, vomiting, diarrhoea and haemorrhaging. In acute cases, even where the correct treatment has been given, death may result within a few hours of the onset of symptoms. Always seek veterinary advice in any cases where this disease may be involved, and ensure that your dog is properly vaccinated against the risks, keeping these vaccinations up to date with yearly booster shots.

Cancer

A term given to a group of diseases. It refers to all malignant tumours and leukaemia, and is quite common in dogs. A tumour is an abnormal swelling, and is not necessarily malignant (progressively worsening and resulting in death if left untreated); if it is not, the tumour is known as benign.

Symptoms

These will depend on the type of the cancer, its location, size and interference with other parts of the dog's body. Many cancers are not detectable by the owner until the cancer is in an advanced state.

Underlying causes

There are many factors that can cause cancer, and these are both environmental and congenital.

A physical examination is one of a number of ways your vet can determine the nature of your dog's illness.

DIAGNOSING CANCER

Physical, X-ray and ultrasound examinations, blood tests and internal examinations (perhaps using an endoscope) are all methods employed by vets to diagnose various cancers.

Owner action

During treatment, it is essential that you follow the vet's advice exactly, ensuring that any drug, diet and exercise regimes are adhered to rigidly. Always discuss any problems or queries with the vet, who will be happy to offer advice and assistance.

COST

Most cancers require long-term treatment involving either high-cost drug therapy or expensive techniques, so the cost for treatment is likely to be high.

Treatment

Treatments vary according to the cause, severity and position of the cancer. It is always better to have any disease treated at an earlier rather than a later stage, if treatment is to have a chance of success.

In chemotherapy, cytotoxic drugs are used. These drugs are designed to kill the cells in the cancer, and are used either in conjunction with surgery, to ensure that no malignant cells remain in the dog's body, or on their own, in cases where it is impossible to remove a malignant tumour surgically.

Radiotherapy is another treatment option. It involves using ionizing radiation, and an optimal dose of this radiation is given to a specific part of the body to destroy the diseased tissue without damaging other parts that are not affected by the disease.

Cushing's disease

Technically known as hyperadrenocorticalism, Cushing's disease occurs when the dog's adrenal glands produce excessive amounts of cortisol, a steroid hormone. There are two adrenal glands, situated near the kidneys. The centre of the glands (the medulla) produces adrenalin, while the outside (the cortex) produces corticosteroids, of which the principal hormone is cortisol. Adrenalin is known as the 'fight or flight' hormone, as it prepares the animal for rapid action. Cortisol controls the water and salt content in the body.

Symptoms

Dogs affected by Cushing's disease may show the following symptoms:
polydipsia (an excessive thirst); polyuria (production of large amounts of urine); swelling of the abdomen (due to an enlarged liver and fluid retention); alopecia on the flanks (see p. 65); coat colour changes; and muscle wasting and general debilitation.

URGENCY INDICATOR

Dogs showing symptoms of Cushing's disease should be taken for veterinary examination as soon as possible.

DIAGNOSING CUSHING'S DISEASE

The vet will need to carry out hormone tests, to determine if Cushing's disease is present. These tests will also reveal the cause of the problem, and therefore the treatment.

Underlying causes

The cause of Cushing's disease is either an adrenal gland tumour, or more commonly a tumour of the pituitary gland.

Owner action

Apart from giving tender loving care and adhering to any treatment regime prescribed by the vet, there is little that you can do.

Treatment

Where the problem is caused by an adrenal tumour, the affected gland may be surgically removed. Where the problem is in the pituitary gland, drug treatment (mitotane) will be given by mouth; this drug is given with food, and the person giving the drug must take care to wear gloves while handling it. Monitoring of the affected dog will be necessary to determine the actual dosage of the drug necessary to achieve the target of treating the polydipsia, that is, reducing the dog's water intake.

COST

Surgery to remove the affected gland(s) will be quite costly, while the extended drug therapy necessary for other forms of treatment is likely to be moderately expensive.

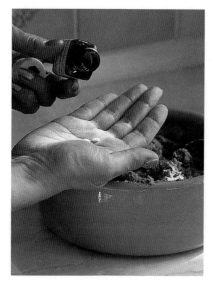

Many pills and other medicines can be given easily in the dog's meal, but you must check that the tablets have indeed been eaten.

Epilepsy

A condition in which a dog suffers from repeated fits or seizures, which are symptoms of abrupt changes in the brain functions of the affected dog.

Symptoms

Convulsions or 'fits', due to violent contractions of muscles, a result of the abnormal electrical activity of the brain. If these seizures are not treated, they will recur at shorter and shorter intervals, eventually leading to status epilepticus, which is continuous seizures.

There are three phases to seizures:
1 The aura – *lasting from a couple of minutes to several days. During this phase, the dog appears agitated and anxious.*
2 The ictus – *the dog passes into unconsciousness. His eyes will be staring, and his legs rigid, quickly followed by 'jaw-champing' and fast paddling actions of the legs. Within a few minutes of this, the dog's breathing will become extremely strenuous.*
3 The post-ictal phase – *the dog's convulsive movements will stop, and his muscles relax. At the same time, his breathing will return to normal, and the dog will regain consciousness. When he has come round, he will appear confused and dazed for up to two days. During this recovery period, the dog may eat far more than normal, bark and cry more, and spend much time pacing around.*
    If a dog suffers partial seizures, which only affect one part of the body, the symptoms may include rapid side-to-side movement of the head, spasms in the legs (sometimes only one leg is affected), or unusual behaviour, such as aggression or even screaming for no apparent reason.

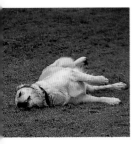

A dog having a seizure must undergo veterinary investigation as soon as possible.

Underlying causes

Disturbances in the dog's central nervous system, resulting from electrical abnormalities in the brain, will result in epilepsy. There are many possible causes of epilepsy, including infections (either viral or bacterial), head injuries, tumours of the brain, hypocalcaemia (low levels of calcium in the dog's blood), hypoglycaemia (abnormally low levels of sugar in the dog's blood), renal (kidney) disease, liver disease or poisoning.

    If a dog is epileptic, he will probably suffer his first seizure between the ages of one and three years. Bitches are less likely to become epileptic than dogs, although bitches who do have seizures are most likely to have them when they are in season. In young dogs and puppies, seizures are usually a symptom of an infection. While any dog could be epileptic, some breeds of dog are more susceptible than others. These include border collie, cocker spaniel, golden retriever, Irish setter, Labrador retriever, miniature schnauzer, poodle, St Bernard and wire-haired terrier.

Owner action

If your dog is fitting, do not touch him, but move any objects around him on which he could injure himself. Keep quiet and, if possible, darken the area. As he comes out of his fit, speak calmly and quietly to your dog to reassure and comfort him. *Never* place a dog that is having a fit in your car and drive him to the veterinary practice; wait until he has recovered and then take him, ensuring that you drive steadily, and do not further upset him. In some cases, it may be necessary for the dog to be kept where he is, and the vet will have to attend him at home.

Treatment

Long-term treatment for epilepsy will involve finding the cause of the problem and treating it. Once this is done, anticonvulsant drugs may be prescribed, but only if the fitting is regular and persistent.

Euthanasia

There comes a time when the kindest thing – for the dog concerned – is for him to be painlessly put to sleep. Reaching that decision can be extremely distressing for the owner and other people concerned, but at all times, the welfare and happiness of the dog must be given priority. All too often, owners postpone the inevitable, often because they cannot bear the thought of being parted from their beloved pet. While this is perfectly understandable, it is also very unfair on the dog.

Euthanasia of domestic dogs is almost always carried out by a vet injecting a powerful anaesthetic directly into the dog's bloodstream, usually via a vein in his foreleg. This causes the dog to become drowsy, lapse into unconsciousness and then die peacefully in just a matter of seconds. The whole process, while

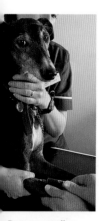

Dogs are usually euthanased with a massive overdose of barbiturate, delivered directly into a vein.

obviously upsetting for the humans involved, particularly the dog's owner, is entirely painless for the dog.

The decision to end a pet's life is the decision of the owner, but it should be based on information and advice from the vet. Ask the vet for details of the condition, and physical and mental state of your dog, and also what the future may hold for the dog if he is not put to sleep. The final decision, however, must be yours. You will never be rushed to make this decision, and you may wish to discuss it with other members of your family. Particularly where children are concerned, it will be necessary to explain to everyone what is going to happen to your dog, in order that no one is under any illusions.

Once the decision has been made, you should spend a little time considering the practicalities. You may wish to have your dog's body cremated or buried, and so will need to make these arrangements before taking your dog on his final visit to the veterinary practice. Many vets will allow the dog's body to remain at the practice until collected by the pet funeral service, and this may help you to cope with your grief over the loss of a loved one. Do not be worried about crying in the surgery; this is perfectly normal and no one will think any the less of you for this action. It often helps to spend a few minutes alone with your dog prior to euthanasia and afterwards, and your vet will respect your wishes.

It is quite normal for the owner of a dog which has been put to sleep to feel sad, angry and guilty. Your vet may offer you counselling. One of the best ways to get over the death of a beloved pet is to be sure that you have acted at all times in the best interests of your dog, and that he has had a good, happy life with you.

Accidents and emergencies

By definition, accidents happen when we least expect them to, so it is wise to be prepared to carry out first aid. Emergency situations require immediate action, and if you are familiar with first aid practice you may be able to limit the injuries suffered by your dog, and in some cases, you may even save his life.

All first aid principles are the same, regardless of whether you are dealing with a person or an animal, and everyone should have a basic training in the subject. Courses are run by first aid organizations throughout the world, and going on such a course may help you to save a life. It is important to practise relevant procedures *before* you encounter an emergency. Most vets will help with this, and will demonstrate the simple procedures necessary. Once you have been shown the procedures, try them out and practise on your dog while he is fit and healthy, and you are under no real pressure. In an emergency situation, you will be under pressure, and that is not the time to try out new procedures for the first time, especially with a dog that may be in severe pain, and therefore less than co-operative.

Your own confidence in an emergency situation will help you to keep calm – vital where the dog's life is, quite literally, in your hands until a trained practitioner can take over from you.

WARNING: NEVER FORGET THAT VETERINARY TREATMENT SHOULD ALWAYS BE SOUGHT FOR A SICK OR AILING DOG.

Quick reference

Emergency techniques
Artificial respiration   104
Chest compression   104
Severe bleeding   105

Serious injuries
The role of the first aider   106
Immediate action in an emergency   106
Specific injuries and conditions   108
Moving and lifting an injured dog   108

Major injuries and dangerous conditions
Bleeding   110
    External   110
    Internal   111
Breathing problems   111
    Choking   111
    Drowning   112
Burns   112
    Heat burns   112
    Chemical burns   113
Electrocution (electric shock)   113
Fits and convulsions   113
Fractures   113
Heatstroke   114
Narcolepsy   114
Poisoning   114
    Types of poisoning   115
Shock   116
Swollen abdomen   117

Minor injuries
Bites and stings   117
    Dog bites   117
    Insect bites   117
    Rat bites   117
    Snake bites   117
Minor bleeding   118
Broken teeth   118
Severe diarrhoea   118
Eye injury   118
Fainting   118
Foreign bodies   119
    In the anus   119
    In the ear   119
    In the eye   119
    In the nose   119
    In a wound   119
Lameness   119
Vomiting   119

The first aid kit   120

Emergency techniques

The basics of first aid are as simple as ABC:

Airways **B**reathing **C**irculation

In other words, in emergency situations, the priority is to clear the dog's airway, to enable him to breathe, and to ensure that the blood is circulating properly, that is, the heart is beating. Then you can deal with any other symptoms.

Artificial respiration

If you find your dog unconscious in a collapsed state, firstly check that he is breathing. Check the colour of the dog's tongue; if there is little or no breathing, the tongue will appear blue/black. If he is not breathing, check for foreign objects lodged in his mouth or throat, blocking his airways. Remove any blockages. Next, extend the dog's neck, by gently lifting up his chin. This will open up the dog's airway. If he is still not breathing, hold his mouth shut, and cover his nose with your mouth. Gently breathe up the dog's nose, giving approximately 30 breaths every minute.

An alternative method of artificial respiration with a small dog is to hold the dog by his hind legs and, keeping your arms straight, swing the dog to the left and then to the right. This transfers the weight of the dog's internal organs on and off the diaphragm, causing the lungs to fill and empty of air. Keep this up until the dog begins breathing on his own, help arrives, or you believe the dog to be beyond help. **Caution** Never try this if you suspect that the dog may have any injury which may be aggravated by using this method.

Chest compression

Next, check for a heartbeat. To do this, put your ear on the dog's chest, on the dog's left-hand side, just behind his elbow. If the heart is beating, you should hear it. You can also check by putting your fingers in the same position. Another method of checking whether the heart is beating is to test for a pulse by placing two fingers on the inside of the dog's thigh, in the groin area.

If no heartbeat is present, you will need to begin chest compressions. The techniques used vary with the size of the injured dog. With small to medium dogs (up to the size of a cocker spaniel), you will need to squeeze the chest with your hands. To do this, place

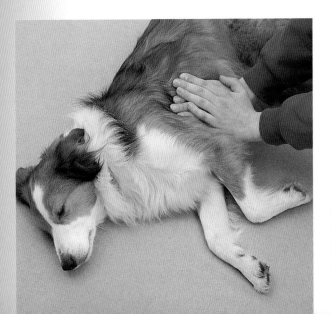

If your dog has no heartbeat, it is essential that chest compressions begin as soon as possible.

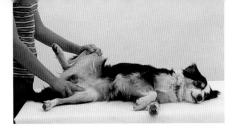

Checking a dog's pulse by placing two fingers on the inner side of the dog's thigh.

one hand on either side of the dog's chest, just behind his elbows, and squeeze the chest in a smooth action, giving two compressions every second. Always use the flat of the hands and never the fingers. Also, be careful not to use too much force, as it is all too easy to break the dog's ribs. With larger dogs, you will need to place both hands on the dog's left-hand side, about level with the dog's elbow. Apply steady pressure at a rate of about two compressions every second.

Never attempt chest compressions if you suspect that the dog may have a chest injury.

Whichever method you use, give two breaths to the dog (artificial respiration) for about every four compressions. You must keep this up until the dog's heart begins to beat, or you cannot physically do any more, or a vet takes over from you. Keep checking for a heartbeat or a pulse throughout your attempts at heart massage.

Severe bleeding

Most people are not used to seeing blood, and so overestimate the amount being lost. It is easy to panic at the sight of blood, but it is important to remain cool, calm and collected.

Bleeding, or haemorrhage, must be controlled once you are certain that the dog is breathing and its heart is beating. Applying pressure, either directly or indirectly, or if the injury is on a limb, raising the limb, will help stem any blood flow. Use gauze, cotton wool or a clean handkerchief or piece of clothing to cover the wound and stem the flow. Direct pressure is simply pressure applied directly to the site of the bleeding, and can be done by squeezing the area in your hand, or holding a piece of cloth firmly to the affected area.

Never apply direct pressure to any wound with an object still impaled in it, or with a piece of bone protruding from it. In such circumstances, you will have to apply indirect pressure, either by applying pressure to the blood vessels above the wound (nearer to the heart) or by making a ring bandage and placing this around the object or bone, holding the ring bandage in place and applying pressure using another bandage or similar. A ring bandage is made by winding a piece of clean cloth (such as a triangular bandage) into a circle; the circle should be slightly larger than the area over which it is to be placed.

Tourniquets must *never* be applied, since they can cut off the blood flow completely, causing severe – often life-threatening – danger to the patient.

The way in which the blood flows out of the wound will give you an idea of the type of blood vessel that is involved. Arteries carry blood from the heart to the organs and tissues. With one exception (the pulmonary artery, which passes blood from heart to lungs), all arteries carry oxygenated blood, which is bright red, whereas the veins, again with one exception (the pulmonary vein, which passes blood from the lungs to the heart) carry de-oxygenated blood, which is very dark. Once the de-oxygenated blood is exposed to the atmosphere, the haemoglobin (which carries the oxygen in the blood) will become enriched with oxygen, thus turning the blood bright red. However, there can be no mistaking the way in which the different blood vessels actually bleed. The arteries carry blood under quite high pressure, as this blood comes directly from the heart. Any blood coming from an artery will therefore spurt out, whereas blood from the veins, under far less pressure, will flow smoothly. The blood vessels between the arteries and the veins, and which pass through organs and the skin, are called capillaries; capillary blood oozes slowly. Arterial blood will flow much faster than the other types, so will need to be attended to earlier. The type of bleeding will also be a good indication of the type and severity of the wound.

Serious injuries

THE ROLE OF THE FIRST AIDER

The priorities of the first aider are to:

● **Sustain life**
● **Prevent the victim's condition worsening**
● **Promote the victim's recovery**
● **Always remember to ensure your own safety at all times**

Immediate action in an emergency

In the event of an accident occurring, the first aider should do the following:

1 Assess the situation

Approach the injured dog carefully, looking for signs of injury and also any signs of danger to yourself or the dog. If the injured dog is in the middle of a road, consider moving him to a position safe for both the dog and yourself. Take care not to aggravate any injuries when moving a dog. Pick him up carefully, not putting any undue pressure on, or pulling, any area which may be injured. It is probably a good idea to fit a muzzle to the dog (see p. 121), as he will be frightened and

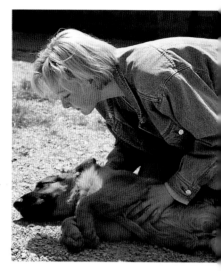

in pain, making him more likely to bite. Speak to the dog throughout in a soft, calm voice, using his name if you know it.

Try to figure out what happened and what injuries the dog has sustained. Ask any witnesses to tell you what happened. This information will help you to decide how to deal with the situation.

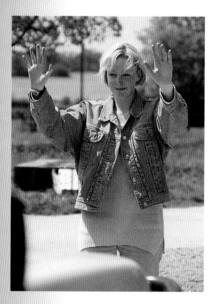

REMEMBER:
You must consider your own safety before attempting a rescue. Never risk your own life to try to save an injured dog, for example by running into a busy road. Always assess the situation before you attempt any rescue or begin any first aid work.

CHECKLIST OF ACTION POINTS

1 Always remember that your own safety is paramount.
2 Assess the situation.
3 Protect yourself and others from injury by the injured dog or traffic.
4 Examine the dog.
5 Diagnose injuries.
6 Treat injuries/treat for pain.
7 Keep the dog warm, calm and quiet.
8 If injuries are serious, contact vet.
9 Protect the dog from further injury.

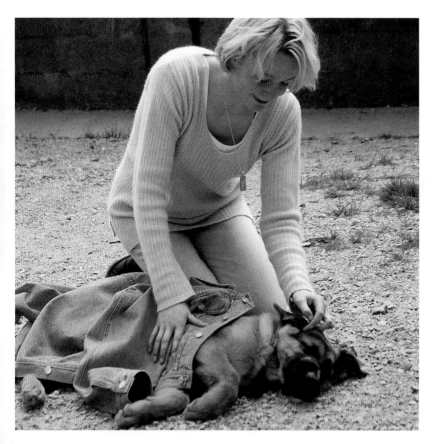

Opposite above: **Examine the dog in situ unless your own safety is compromised by so doing.**

Opposite below: **If the dog is involved in a road traffic accident and is still on the road, you must stop the traffic while the dog is removed to a place that is safe for both you and the dog.**

Left: **Offer the dog soothing words, using his name, to keep him calm until assistance arrives.**

2 Diagnose the dog's condition

If the dog is unconscious, gently shake him and, if you do not get a response, pinch his ear. If there is still no reaction, the dog really is unconscious, and not merely stunned. Look at his chest to see if he is breathing; if he is not, you must get him breathing (see p. 104). You must then check that he has a heartbeat and if not, carry out chest compressions (see p. 104). If he is breathing, consider whether he will require veterinary treatment, and if so, arrange for the vet to be contacted. You can always take the vet's advice on the situation, but do not allow this action to delay any life-saving actions that may be needed.

3 Examine the dog

Check for any obvious injury, and make a note of its relative seriousness.

Check for bleeding, and treat accordingly (immediately and adequately, p. 105 and 110). Check for any fractures, and treat accordingly (immediately and adequately, see p. 113).

Check for any burns, and treat accordingly (immediately and adequately, see p. 112).

Check the back of the dog's neck for 'lumps' and swellings. Any such lumps may indicate a broken bone, or swelling caused by injury. These symptoms will need to be passed on to the attending vet.

Finally, wait for the vet.

Specific injuries and conditions

Remember: an injured dog may object to being handled or even touched, and so you must be in a position to restrain him correctly (see p. 121).

BURNS:
Minimize the damage from burns by cooling the burned area as quickly as possible with water (see p. 112)

OPEN WOUNDS:
These must be covered with clean dressings to reduce the risk of infection.

UNCONSCIOUS DOG:
Check for breathing and keep the airways open (see p. 104)

FRACTURES:
Prevent further damage from broken bones by immobilizing the affected limb to avoid further movement and injury. (see p. 113)

BODY TEMPERATURE:
It is extremely important that an injured dog is kept warm. If you have a 'space blanket', the dog should be wrapped in this. Failing a proper space blanket, use a sheet of 'bubble wrap', a coat or a jacket. If the dog is losing heat at a fast rate, or the surrounding temperature is extremely low, and it is necessary to try to warm up the injured dog, then you can snuggle up to it, sharing your own body heat with the dog. Never do this if there is any risk of the dog attacking you, unless you have taken the relevant precautions, such as fitting a muzzle on the dog (see p. 121).

Moving and lifting an injured dog

You should not move any injured dog unless you have to, as any movement may aggravate his injuries. However, if you do need to move him, you should do this with great care. Lifting a large dog, such as a Labrador or German shepherd, using the wrong technique, will put both yourself and the dog at risk of injury.

It is much easier to restrain, examine or treat a dog at about waist height, and so, if possible, the dog should be placed on a table or bench. First cover the surface of the table with a blanket or towel to help prevent the dog from slipping, which may cause him to panic. Lift him onto the elevated surface using the techniques demonstrated in the photographs. Once the dog is on the table, use one hand to hold him firmly by the collar, if he is wearing one, and if not, place one arm around the dog's neck, unless this will aggravate his injuries. Place the other arm over the dog's back and under his chest, and you should be able to hold him firmly and safely.

Throughout any restraint, you must be firm but kind: talk quietly and calmly to the dog, offering him reassurance, and never frighten him by using too much force. To help ensure that your dog will always be fairly easy to restrain, practise restraint on him throughout his life, starting when he is a young puppy.

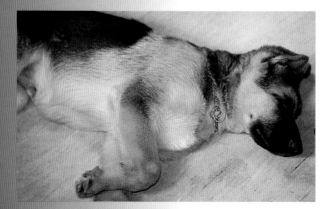

Try not to move an injured dog, as any movement may cause further damage.

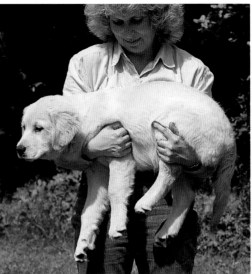

The correct way to carry a small dog, supporting his weight evenly.

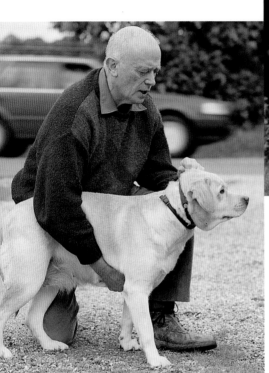

Restraining a dog by holding his collar while keeping one arm around his abdomen will ensure that he will not panic.

LIFTING A DOG

1 Kneel close to the dog, and place one arm under his chest, in front of his front legs, embracing the dog's chest.
2 Place your other arm under the dog's rump, and angle your hands towards each other.
3 Keeping your back straight, stand up, keeping the dog's weight on your chest.
4 If the dog is of a large breed, you may need help to lift him.
5 A home-made stretcher is an excellent way of moving a large, unconscious dog, although this will require two people to carry it. If you are on your own, roll the injured dog onto a blanket, coat or similar, and drag him.

MOVING AN INJURED DOG

1 Cover the surface of the table with a towel or similar to help prevent the dog from slipping.
2 Lift the dog onto the table, using a safe lifting technique.
3 Hold the dog by his collar with one hand, and place the other arm across the dog's back and under his chest to hold him securely.
4 If this is done correctly, the dog will not be able to lunge forward, turn his head from side to side, or move his head up or down to attack anyone.
5 If the dog's injuries are best treated with him lying down, then you must place him in the lying position on the table, and then restrain him. Using safe lifting techniques, start with the dog standing on the table.
6 Reaching over his back, take hold of the dog's legs on the side nearest to you. Hold them firmly just above the knees.
7 As the dog leans into you, slowly move his legs away from your body; this will cause him to slide down on to the surface of the table.
8 When he is lying down on the table, move your hands to grasp both pairs of legs: the front pair in one hand and the rear pair in the other hand. By lowering your elbows, you can restrain the dog's head with one, and his backside with the other, ensuring that he cannot move. It is vital that you do not place your body weight on the dog.

Major injuries and dangerous conditions

Bleeding

EXTERNAL
There are several different types of wound that a dog may suffer, and each requires slightly different treatment.

Minor wounds:
See p. 117 for the treatment of minor wounds.

Major wounds:
Clean (incised) cuts These are straight cuts, like one from a sharp knife blade. Bleeding, which may be profuse, helps clean the wound of debris, and this lessens the possibility of infection. Very often, incised cuts will bleed very little, if at all, even though the cut may be very deep, because the cut has not affected any major blood vessel. Any incised cut affecting the toes or a limb may cause damage to tendons, and so veterinary treatment should be sought. Many minor incised cuts will heal on their own, once they have been cleaned.

If possible, bleeding from an incised cut should be stemmed by direct pressure; if this is not possible, apply indirect pressure on an artery at the heart side of the wound. To find the artery, feel along the affected area, and you will be able to feel the vessel under the dog's skin. Elevating the injury will enable gravity to help reduce the blood flow. Apply a suitable dressing. Large and/or deep cuts will almost certainly require sutures (stitches) from a vet.

Lacerated cuts These are tears in the skin, such as those caused by barbed wire, for example, and bleed less profusely than incised cuts.

Puncture (stab) wounds Puncture wounds, which can be caused by nails, slivers of wood and other such objects, usually appear very

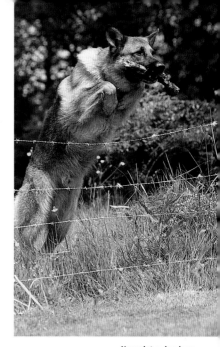

Never let a dog leap over barbed wire fencing, since this can result in horrific injuries.

small at the surface but, of course, could be very deep. *Never* remove any object from a wound, as this may aggravate the injury and/or allow large amounts of bleeding (while in place, such an object acts as a plug, and may be preventing massive blood loss). Apply pressure around the wound site, using a dressing to maintain the pressure, and seek veterinary advice immediately.

Gunshot wounds If you have a working gun-dog, he may be accidentally shot. The most common type of wound to a working dog is from a shotgun, in which case the dog will be peppered with balls of shot (pellets), which will all require removal; bleeding should not be profuse. The vet will need to take an X-ray of the dog in order to locate all the pellets.

The other type of gunshot wound is from a bullet. Bullets make two wounds – an entry wound on the way in and an exit wound going out. Where 'sporting' (hollow point) ammunition is used, the exit wound will be several times larger than the entry wound. Where the bullet passes through any part(s) of the dog's anatomy, damage may be inflicted on any organ or tissue with which it comes into contact, and so all such wounds must be referred to a vet immediately. In the unlikely event that the bullet does not exit, there will only be an entry hole. Your vet may use X-ray examinations to find the bullet inside the dog's body, and the bullet will then be surgically removed.

In all cases of gunshot wounds, stem the flow of blood, keep the dog calm, checking for signs of trauma, and seek veterinary treatment immediately.

INTERNAL

Internal injuries are often manifested by swellings and bruising (contusions) in the dog's abdomen, neck or any limb. Bleeding from the dog's mouth, eyes, ears, nose, anus or sex organs is another sign of internal injuries. A careful watch must be kept on the injured dog. Any dog that is showing any of these signs, or any signs of shock (see p. 116) must be taken to a vet as soon as possible. Sometimes, the stools of a dog suffering internal bleeding will be very dark reddish-brown.

You should always remember that the most common causes of bleeding from a bitch's vulva are oestrus and cystitis (see p. 33); oestrus, of course, does not require veterinary treatment. Likewise, in the male dog, a common cause of bleeding from the penis is prostate problems (see p. 78), and this will not require emergency treatment in the same way that an internal injury would. However, any bleeding from the penis should be examined by a vet, just in case.

Breathing problems

If your dog has stopped breathing, perform artificial respiration, see p. 104.

Dogs gasping for breath are obviously showing symptoms of some form of breathing difficulty; this may be heatstroke, fluid on the lungs or an obstruction of some kind blocking the airway.

If the dog is suffering from heatstroke, he will appear very distressed, restless, and will pant a lot. If left untreated, his condition will rapidly deteriorate; he will drool and appear to be drunk, staggering around and completely unsteady on his feet. The treatment is to cool the dog down (see p. 114).

Choking:

Sometimes, a dog's breathing problems may be caused by something very simple, the most obvious cause being a blockage of the mouth or throat. Typically, such a blockage may be caused by a piece of wood broken or bitten off a branch thrown by the dog's owner for it to fetch. I recommend that owners *do not* throw sticks for their dogs to fetch. There are plenty of toys that are designed to be thrown for the dog to fetch back safely.

If your dog suddenly appears to be choking, you must act immediately. To try to get him to a veterinary practice will waste time,

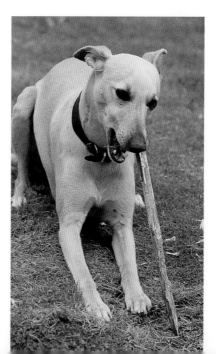

Many dogs choke on pieces of wood that their owner has thrown for them to fetch.

and may result in his death. Take a secure hold on him (put him on his lead if at all possible), and open his mouth to look inside and see if he has anything stuck in there. It is important that you have a good look in the dog's mouth before you start putting your fingers inside, as you may make matters worse by pushing a foreign object further down the throat. Very often, you will require assistance to remove an object blocking the dog's mouth, so that one of you can hold open the mouth to reduce the risk of the other being bitten. *Never* attempt to remove an object wedged in the dog's throat.

If you cannot remove the foreign object, you will need to take further, more drastic action. Holding the dog's hind legs, lift them over your knees, holding them between your knees. Placing one hand on either side of the chest, squeeze using jerky movements, making the dog 'cough'. Take care that you apply pressure proportional to the size of the dog: little pressure on a small puppy, more for a large adult dog. Squeeze about 5–6 times and the dog should cough out the lodged object.

Once the foreign object has been removed, you must let your dog rest, and take him to the vet for a check-up.

If the foreign object is in the dog's throat or you cannot remove it from the mouth easily, obtain veterinary assistance urgently.

Drowning:
It is good practice to prevent your dog from entering any water without you telling him to. He should never be allowed to swim in fast-flowing rivers, stagnant ponds or any water that may have been polluted, and he should never be encouraged to run over iced-up ponds, as there is a risk of him falling through the ice and then not being able to get out of the water.

If your dog gets into difficulties while swimming, ensure your own safety before making any rescue attempts. Once he has been pulled from the water, he should be held upside down (if possible) to allow the water to drain from his lungs. If your dog is too big or heavy for you to attempt this, try to lift his back end, for example by resting his back legs over a seat or fence.

Your dog will need veterinary treatment, and so someone should contact the vet as soon as possible. If you are on your own at the time of the emergency, shout to attract attention, and then ask anyone answering your calls to contact your vet immediately and explain the situation.

Check that your dog is breathing. If he is not, you must begin artificial respiration, then check for a heartbeat and, if necessary, carry out chest compressions (see p. 104). If luck is on your side, your dog should begin coughing and spluttering. Keep him quiet and calm. Rub him to dry off some of the water, and wrap him in a blanket or coat to keep him warm on his way to the vet.

Burns

There are two types of burn, one caused by heat and the other caused by chemicals.

Heat burns:
The first treatment for any burn caused by heat, including scalds, is to reduce the heat, that is, cool the burn. This is best achieved by pouring cold water on the affected area. If you can stand the dog in a bath, run cold water on the affected area for at least ten minutes. The cooling will reduce the pain and the severity of the burn. If you can get the injured dog into the garden, use a hose pipe to douse the affected area thoroughly with cold water. Do not use the hose pipe at full power, or apply too much cold water at once, because too sudden a drop in the dog's temperature may cause more serious problems; his temperature should therefore be reduced gradually.

While you are cooling the burned area, get someone to arrange for you to see the vet as soon as possible. Once you have cooled the affected area for at least ten minutes, cover the wound with a clean damp cloth and wrap the injured dog in a space blanket or equivalent to keep him warm. If possible, get someone else to drive you to the vet, while you stay in the rear seat with the dog, to keep him calm and prevent him aggravating his injury.

Chemical burns:

In the case of chemical burns, there is a grave danger of the dog ingesting the chemical if he licks the affected area, burning the inside of his mouth and throat etc. To help prevent this, apply a muzzle to the dog as soon as possible. Wear rubber gloves to ensure that the chemical does not injure you. Once the dog is muzzled, thoroughly wash the affected area with running water, either by placing the dog in the bath and running water over the burn, or by using a hose pipe in the garden.

While you are washing the affected area, get someone to arrange for you to see the vet as soon as possible. Once you have washed the affected area for at least ten minutes, cover the wound with a clean damp cloth and wrap the injured dog in a space blanket or equivalent to keep him warm. If possible, get someone else to drive you to the vet, while you stay in the rear seat with the dog, to keep him calm and prevent him from licking the affected area or aggravating his injury.

Electrocution (electric shock)

A big danger in treating dogs that have been electrocuted is the threat to the first aider. It is easy to rush in without considering any danger you might be in.

Whenever you suspect that a dog has been electrocuted, ensure that the power is switched off *before* you approach the injured dog. If it is not possible to switch off the

power, do not approach the dog.

Once the power has been switched off, and you are no longer in any danger, check that the dog is breathing. If it is not, begin artificial respiration, as detailed on p. 104.

Electrocution will almost inevitably cause burns, which will need treating (see p. 112), but they should only be considered after the dog is breathing normally, as they are unlikely to be life-threatening.

Fits and convulsions

Fits, convulsions and seizures are all the same, and are not a disease, but are symptoms of an underlying problem. There are many possible causes for convulsions, one of the most common in dogs being heatstroke (see p. 114) her causes include poisoning, an infection of some kind, genetic disorders, brain defects (for example, distemper or even rabies), shock (trauma), liver disorders, kidney disorders or many other medical problems. Although rarely seen, young puppies suffering from a heavy infestation of roundworms may also show symptoms of fits. If a dog suffers regular, repeated fits, this may indicate that he is in fact suffering from epilepsy (see p. 100).

Do not attempt to hold down a fitting dog, but take care to limit how far the dog can move. If your dog is suffering from convulsions, you should seek urgent medical attention for him, as seizures are extremely serious, and potentially life-threatening.

Fractures

Fractures (see p. 46) are caused by either direct or indirect pressure on the bones, which may crack or actually break. Where the bone is broken and pierces the skin, this is known as an open or compound fracture; others are called closed fractures. Signs of such injury are obvious – painful movement of the limb, tenderness, swelling, loss of control of

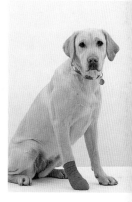

A fractured leg will need dressing and support.

the limb, deformity of the limb, unnatural movement of the limb, and crepitus (the sensation or, in very bad cases, the sound of the two ends of the bones grinding on each other).

Keep the patient quiet, and steady and support the injured limb, immobilizing it with bandages and splints if necessary, to prevent it moving and causing greater damage. Use any suitable object available for splinting, such as a piece of wood or a plastic ruler, and place it on the affected limb on the opposite side to any open wound. Tie the splint in place with a bandage, if available, or a tie or even tights or stockings may be used. Raising the limb will help reduce discomfort and swelling (by reducing the blood flow).

Heatstroke

Dogs cannot tolerate high temperatures and may die from heatstroke. Prevention is better than cure. Where you position your dog's kennel is very important, and it is also vital to remember that inside a car the temperature can quickly rise to a dangerous level, even in the cooler sunshine of autumn and spring. If you leave your dog in a car for any period of time, particularly when the surrounding temperature is high and/or there is a lot of sunshine, your dog may be dead on your return. No animal should be left unattended in a vehicle, or transported in full sunlight, without adequate ventilation. You must always remember that the sun does not stay in the same position throughout the day, so even if your car is in the shade when you leave it, it may be in full sun later on. In extreme summer temperatures, or in areas where it is known that temperatures will be high, even more care must be taken than normal.

The first sign of heatstroke or heat exhaustion is an agitated dog in obvious distress. Affected dogs may stretch out and pant heavily. The affected dog will start to drool and stagger around as if drunk; if left untreated, the dog will eventually collapse, pass into a coma and die.

Immediately a dog shows symptoms of heatstroke, you must act fast; delay can be fatal. The dog's body is overheating, so your first task is to lower his body temperature. With mildly affected dogs, simply moving them to a cool area, and ensuring a steady passage of cool air over them, is usually effective. Light spraying with cold water from a plant mister is also beneficial. If the dog is only suffering a mild case of heatstroke, once he has started to recover, ensure that he is thoroughly dried and placed in a cool area to recover fully.

In bad cases, a hose pipe (on a fine misting spray) in the garden is effective. In very bad cases, cover the affected dog with wet blankets (making sure that the mouth and nose are clear), and keep dousing the blankets with cold water to keep them wet. Seek veterinary advice for all dogs badly affected by heatstroke.

In all cases of heatstroke, it is vital to keep the head cool, as the brain may be quite literally cooked and brain death can occur.

Narcolepsy

A dog suffering from narcolepsy will appear to be extremely sleepy, although he will not lose consciousness. The condition is often associated with a condition known as cataplexy, where the affected dog will collapse and refuse to move. Some rat poisons also have this effect on a dog.

If your dog shows any of these signs, consult the vet as soon as possible.

Poisoning

In cases of poisoning, it is most important to discover which poison your dog has taken. In the United Kingdom, with COSHH (Control of Substances Hazardous to Health) regulations, manufacturers must provide details of all substances that may be ingested. Businesses must also keep all such details of all substances that they use, on the premises. Seek veterinary advice immediately in all cases of suspected poisoning, giving details of the poison that your dog has ingested if you know what it is. This will allow the practice time to get the relevant information from the manufacturer.

Do *not* make your dog vomit unless the manufacturer gives specific guidelines to do so. If you are instructed to make the dog vomit, place a couple of washing soda (sodium carbonate) crystals on the back of the dog's tongue. If you have no washing soda, use mustard or salt in a strong solution. It is pointless to induce vomiting in a dog that has ingested a poison more than four hours earlier, as the substance will have passed through the stomach.

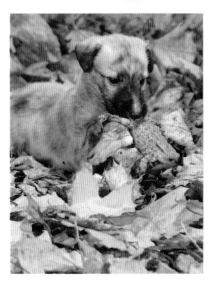

Above: **Dogs can easily come into contact with poisonous substances which are in everyday use in the human home.**

Left: **Dogs cannot resist catching toads, and may be poisoned as a consequence.**

TYPES OF POISONING

Corrosive acids Car battery acid and the descaler used in central heating systems and kettles etc. are examples of corrosive acids. The acid must be neutralized as soon as possible, and the best way to do this is to get the dog to drink a solution of bicarbonate of soda (baking soda). The solution should be made up of half a teaspoon (approximately 2.5 ml) of sodium bicarbonate, dissolved in 250 ml (8 fl oz) of water. The sodium bicarbonate will dissolve better if the water is warm.
Never induce vomiting with corrosive acids.

Corrosive alkalis Creosote (used to treat fences and wooden kennels etc.) is the most common type of corrosive alkali likely to be ingested by a dog. Others may include paint stripper and oven cleaning fluids.

Again, the substance needs to be neutralized, by giving an acid solution (vinegar or orange juice) by mouth. Dilute the vinegar with an equal amount of water, though the orange juice can be given as it is.
Never induce vomiting with corrosive alkalis.

Irritants Irritants with which your dog may come into contact, and thus eat and ingest, include poisonous plants such as laburnum and poinsettia, or chemicals such as arsenic or lead. An extremely common source of dogs suffering from 'poisoning', and one where they will be salivating profusely, is when the dog tries to eat a toad (*Bufo bufo*). The toad's skin is covered with pustules containing toxins designed to protect the creature from predators, and these toxins will affect the dog. Consult a vet immediately.

Narcotics Narcotic substances induce insensibility or stupor. Turpentine, paraffin and human sleeping tablets come under this category. Induce vomiting immediately if you have actually witnessed your dog eating narcotics, but if you are not certain when he may have

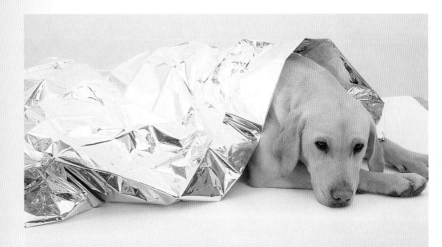

A 'space blanket' will help prevent too much heat loss from an injured or ill dog.

eaten the substance, *do not induce vomiting*. If the narcotic has been in the dog's system for some time, it may be affecting his swallowing reflex, and if so, he may inhale his own vomit, with serious consequences.

If at all possible, keep the affected dog awake until he can be treated by a vet.

Convulsants Convulsants cause fits, which are involuntary actions of voluntary muscles. Slug pellets are the most likely convulsant for a dog to have ingested, but he may have eaten laurel or anti-freeze (ethylene glycol). If you know that your dog has definitely taken these substances, induce vomiting immediately, and seek veterinary guidance and advice.

Shock

Shock, which is an acute fall in blood pressure, is often evident after the dog has been involved in an accident or has been injured; certain diseases can also cause this condition. The symptoms of shock include cool skin, pale lips and gums (due to the lack of circulation); faint, rapid pulse; staring but unseeing eyes.

The dog must be kept warm and the blood circulation returned to normal as soon as possible. Massaging the dog will help to improve his circulation, and wrapping him in a towel or blanket will help keep him warm. The affected dog should be kept quiet and warm, and veterinary treatment sought as soon as possible.

Swollen abdomen

A dog that seems bloated and repeatedly attempts to vomit, but does not produce anything, may be suffering from a very serious affliction known as gastric dilation volvulus complex. This is seen mostly in breeds with big, deep chests (such as Rottweilers). The condition is thought to be triggered (usually) by overeating, and a loop of the intestine forms and blocks the digestive tract. Seek immediate veterinary treatment, or the dog may die.

Minor Injuries

Bites and stings

There are four types of bite and sting: dog, insect, rat and snake.

DOG BITES

Dogs are more likely to suffer from bites from other dogs than from any other animal, especially if allowed to wander, unsupervised, in public places. Such dogs are regularly involved in fights with other dogs.

Before attempting to break up a fight between two or more dogs, ensure your own safety. A long-handled sweeping brush or broom will help drive off the other dogs, and also keep them far enough away from you to prevent you being bitten. If to hand, a bucket of cold water, or water sprayed from a hose pipe, will help stop the dogs from fighting and give you the opportunity to control them.

If a bite has caused only minor injuries, the area of the bite should be clipped of hair, ensuring that the clippings do not become entangled in the wound itself. Wetting the scissors is recommended, as the hairs stick to the blades rather than falling onto the wound; dipping the scissors into a jug of water after each snip will remove all hairs from the metal. The wound should then be thoroughly washed with a saline solution followed by an antiseptic liquid. Finally, give the area a good dusting with an antiseptic wound powder. If action is not taken, the wound may develop an abscesses.

INSECT BITES (including stings)

Clip a little fur away from the area, so that you can actually see the problem, then wash with saline solution. Bees leave their sting in the victim, wasps do not. If there is a sting present, it should be carefully removed with tweezers and then the area wiped with cotton wool (or a cotton bud) soaked in alcohol, such as surgical spirit. For wasp stings, a little vinegar will prove beneficial while for bee stings, use a little bicarbonate of soda (the stings are alkaline, and the vinegar or bicar-

bonate of soda neutralizes the effect). Dry the area thoroughly, and apply a wet compress to help reduce the irritation and swelling.

Bites and stings in/on the throat can cause swelling that may block the airways and kill the dog; seek veterinary attention urgently.

RAT BITES

Rat bites are some of the most dangerous bites that a dog may suffer. Rats can carry many harmful diseases and their teeth are dirty, so the wounds will become infected.

The area of the wound should be clipped of fur, then cleaned with a saline solution and then an antiseptic liquid; dry and apply liberal amounts of antibiotic dusting powder. Take your dog to the vet as soon as possible, where the vet may administer antibiotics.

SNAKE BITES

There are many venomous snakes, although only one species, the adder (*Vipera berus*) lives in the UK. It is unusual for dogs to be bitten by these reptiles but it does happen.

During the spring or early summer, snakes are rather lethargic, especially the gravid (pregnant) females; this is due to the cool temperatures, since snakes are exothermic and require external heat to warm their bodies to their preferred body temperature. At such times, while they are warming themselves, they will keep still for as long as possible, even when approached. If your dog does not see a snake and stands on it, the snake will bite.

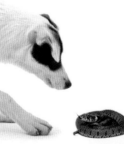

A dog bitten by a venomous snake will require veterinary examination.

CLIPPING OF HAIR AROUND WOUNDS

1. Using scissors with curved blades and rounded ends, and that have been dipped in water, carefully clip the fur around the wound. The clipped fur will stick to the blades of the scissors, preventing any from falling into the wound.
2. Dip the blades of the scissors in the bowl of water, and the clippings will come off in the water.

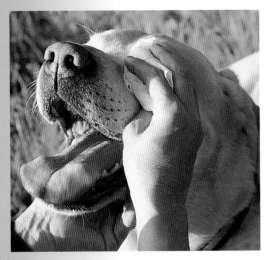

All eye injuries must be seen by a vet as soon as possible after the injury has been sustained.

It is most important that you keep the injured dog as calm as possible and prevent him from running around, or even making any movements, as this will speed up the circulation of the venom around the dog's body. You must also remain calm yourself, as your actions will influence the dog. Seek immediate veterinary attention.

Minor bleeding

The big danger with any cuts is that the injury will have pushed dirt and debris into the wound, and unless there is a great deal of bleeding the dirt will not be washed out. Clean the wound with saline solution (two teaspoonfuls (approximately 10 ml) of salt to 1 litre (1¾ pints) of warm water), dry it, apply an antiseptic ointment or cream, and apply a dressing if necessary.

Broken teeth

Dogs, like humans, can damage their teeth, making eating an extremely painful business (see p. 24). Broken teeth are often accompanied by bleeding from the dog's mouth. They must be treated by the vet.

Severe diarrhoea

Every reader will recognize the signs of diarrhoea, and also realize that this may simply be a symptom of over-eating. However, it may also be a symptom of more serious problems (see p. 32).

In all cases of severe diarrhoea, where over-eating is definitely not the cause, you should prevent your dog eating anything and contact the vet. It is essential that your dog is provided with ample drinking water or, even better, give him re-hydrating fluid (see p. 33). Keep your dog where you can see him, covering the floor with newspapers or similar, and note the times of his motions, and also the consistency, colour and quantity of the diarrhoea. This will help the vet to find the cause of the sudden diarrhoea.

Eye injury

Any injury to the eye can cause serious damage to the dog's sight, so any eye injuries must be seen by the vet (see pp. 16–21).

If your dog has an injured eye he will be holding it half closed, and the eye itself will be swollen and/or bleeding. The dog will probably be trying to rub his affected eye, and this should not be allowed, as it may aggravate the injury. See p. 119 for how to deal with foreign objects in the eye.

If the eye is swollen, the application of a cold compress (a cold wet cloth) may help. Do *not* apply any bandage or compress if you suspect there may be a foreign body in the eye, as this may cause further damage.

Fainting

This is a loss of consciousness caused by a sudden lack of blood supply to the brain. Fainting can also be caused by low blood sugar levels. To treat fainting, clear the dog's airways (see 104) and wait until he is conscious again, checking that the airways remain open. Once he is back on his feet, give the dog gentle walking exercise until he has totally recovered. If you have access to ice or very cold water, it will help your dog if this is applied to his head and his mouth. If fainting recurs frequently, consult the vet.

Foreign bodies

Most dogs are inquisitive, and tend to lead lifestyles that make them prone to picking up items that they really should not, so foreign bodies are quite common in various parts of their anatomy.

IN THE ANUS

A dog that has swallowed a foreign object that his body cannot digest will pass the object out of his anus. Often, this occurs without any problem, and without the owner even knowing about it. Occasionally, however, the object may be seen hanging half out of the anus; the owner must attempt to remove the object without hurting the dog. As most dogs do not take well to interference in this area, it is wise to fit a muzzle to the dog before you start to try to remove the foreign object. It is also extremely helpful if you can get someone to assist you, by firmly but kindly restraining the dog (see p. 121).

Once the dog is muzzled and restrained, carefully examine the foreign object and, unless it appears sharp, gently pull it. If there is any resistance to your pulls, stop immediately, and take the dog to the vet for help.

IN THE EAR

A foreign object in your dog's ear usually leads to the dog shaking his head violently. Look in his ear (in breeds such as spaniels, the ear flap will need to be lifted), but do not attempt to remove anything wedged in the ear canal. Seek immediate veterinary advice.

IN THE EYE

The dog will probably be trying to rub his affected eye, and this should not be allowed, as it may aggravate the injury, so you must physically restrain him.

Holding the dog's head very steady, and using a magnifying lens, look in the eye for any foreign object (such as a grass seed or small piece of hay). Often, such objects get stuck behind the eyelid (either upper or lower). This operation is best if carried out away from bright lights, and with the assistance of a friend.

If any foreign object is seen, do not try to remove it with fingers, tweezers or similar objects, as this may lead to serious and irreparable eye damage. Instead, use warm water, and gently and slowly pour it over the affected eye, while the eyelids are held open. This action may flush out the object.

IN THE NOSE

Unless you are certain that the foreign object is very short, do not attempt to remove it from your dog's nose. Contact the vet immediately.

IN A WOUND

Never remove any foreign object from a wound. To do so may aggravate the wound, and cause further bleeding. Seek veterinary treatment.

Lameness

A dog that is unable to bear his weight on one or more of his legs, or is unable to walk, is described as lame. The condition is covered in detail on p. 40.

If your dog suddenly becomes lame, contact the vet as soon as possible, and keep the dog still and resting until he can be examined.

Vomiting

Vomiting is a muscular reflex action, resulting in expulsion, under force, of the contents of the dog's stomach and/or small intestine (see p. 30). It is quite normal for a dog to vomit small amounts occasionally, and only if the dogs vomits two or three times within a short period should you consult the vet.

If this does occur, prevent your dog from eating or drinking anything, and contact the vet. Keep your dog where you can see him, and note the times of vomiting, the consistency, colour and quantity of the vomit. By doing this, you will help the vet to find the cause of the sudden vomiting.

The first aid kit

Some of the most common dog injuries – minor cuts and abrasions – occur when the dog is going about its daily routine, or is being worked, as with a gundog, and it is important that they are treated as soon as possible, in order to minimize adverse effects on the dog. In order to do this, a small first aid kit should be kept near the kennel or wherever your dog is housed, and taken along on every outing. You should, of course, also have the necessary skill and experience to treat these minor injuries, and you can get advice from your vet on various minor procedures. If there is any doubt as to the seriousness of the injuries, or the dog's general condition, consult the vet as soon as possible: he or she will be happy to advise you on the best course of action.

Contents of a canine first aid kit

A good first aid kit can save much money at the vet's – and may even save your dog's life. It is, however, vital that you know exactly how to use all the items. A good book such as this one is also useful, and should be kept close to the first aid kit.

The following are all items that should be included in a first aid kit, which you should have near at hand at all times. Do not forget to replace any item you use straight away, before it is needed again. Many of the items listed in this kit can be used on either canine or human injuries.

1 ADHESIVE PLASTERS
For applying directly to small wounds and for keeping dressings in place, although the dog will soon chew these off. They can also be used for minor splinting. Try to obtain the special 'non-sticky' plaster that can be purchased from vets and pharmacists as this does not adhere to hair.

2 ALCOHOL (surgical spirits)
For the removal of ticks etc. (see p. 68).

3 ANTIHISTAMINE
For the treatment of insect stings. It comes as cream or lotion, and can be purchased from the vet or a pharmacy.

4 ANTISEPTIC LOTION
For cleaning cuts, wounds and abrasions. Soap and water or brine (salt and water solution made with 2 teaspoonfuls (10 ml) salt to 1 litre (1¾ pints) of water) is as good as antiseptic lotion.

5 BANDAGES
For binding broken limbs and wounds. Keep a selection of small bandages. They will only be temporary, as the dog will chew them off.

6 COTTON BUDS
For cleaning wounds and applying ointments etc. With care, they can also be used to clean the ear flaps but *under no circumstances* should you poke these (or any other object) into the ear canal.

7 COTTON WOOL
For cleaning wounds, cuts and abrasions, and for stemming the flow of blood. Dampen all cotton wool before use with tap water, otherwise strands will stick to the wound, possibly causing complications.

8 ELIZABETHAN COLLAR
Useful to (try to!) prevent a dog from interfering with dressings, sutures etc. It is simple to make one of these using an old plastic bucket by splitting it and cutting a hole in the centre, of a size to fit comfortably around the dog's neck. You could also use a piece of strong cardboard.

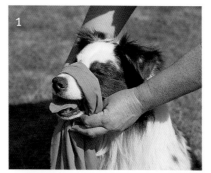

9 EYE WASH

For washing out debris from a dog's eyes. This is particularly useful if you have a working dog that may be regularly pushing through foliage. It is also advisable to obtain some local anaesthetic, sold at pharmacists for relieving the pain of eye injuries, until veterinary treatment can be obtained for the injured dog.

10 KAOLIN PECTATE

For use in cases of diarrhoea. Available from any vet, a pharmacy or even from many supermarkets. Follow the dosage recommendations on the label. Veterinary advice will be given when it is dispensed.

11 KY JELLY

A lubricant that should be applied to the thermometer before it is inserted into the dog's rectum. It is available from a pharmacist or a vet. If KY jelly is not available, petroleum jelly or even liquid soap or washing-up liquid may be used.

12 MUZZLE

No matter how tame you believe your dog to be, when it is in pain it may bite anyone who comes close, particularly when that person is handling the injured area. It is best always to muzzle any injured dog before beginning examination or treatment, although you must never fit a muzzle to any dog that is unconscious, experiencing breathing problems, or has any injuries to his muzzle or jaw.

There are several different types of muzzle available to dog owners. All types of muzzle are available in different sizes, to suit the specific breed and size of dog, and it is important that the correct size is used, if the muzzle is to work effectively. The safest type to fit to an injured dog is the 'classic' type, that forms a cage around the dog's face and is held in

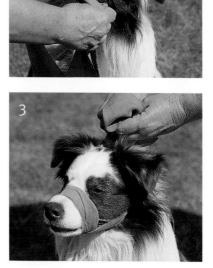

MAKING A MAKESHIFT MUZZLE

1 With a friend assisting by restraining the dog, make a loop around the dog's muzzle (nose), and knot it under the chin.
2 Take the two ends of the tie, and pass them around the dog's neck, under the dog's ears.
3 Tie the material securely, but not too tightly, at the back of the dog's neck, checking that the muzzle is not too tight. Throughout your treatment and transportation of the injured dog, you must watch him for any sign of vomiting. If this happens, remove the muzzle immediately, and do not replace it until the dog has finished vomiting, and you have checked that his airways are clear.

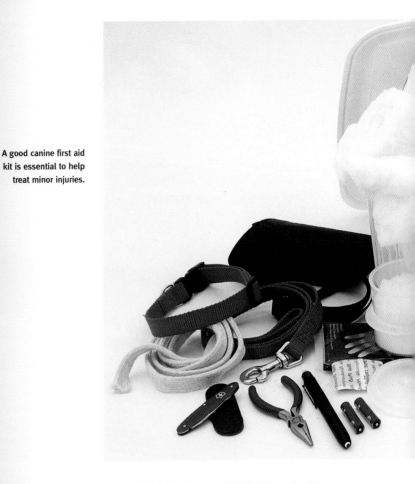

A good canine first aid kit is essential to help treat minor injuries.

place by a strap or straps around the back of the dog's head and/or neck. It completely encases the dog's mouth, preventing it from biting, and the dog can vomit without any risk of inhaling the vomit.

If you do not have a muzzle to hand in an emergency, it is possible to make a temporary muzzle using a bandage, tie, belt, scarf, length of string, or even the dog's own lead (see p. 121).

13 NAIL CLIPPERS

For trimming the dog's nails. These should be top quality. Use the type that work on the guillotine principle, where one blade hits the other, rather than on the scissors principle, which can result in nails being pulled out (see photograph).

14 RECTAL THERMOMETER

For taking the dog's temperature. Modern thermometers are electronic, making a 'beep' when they have been in position long enough to take the dog's temperature, and they have a digital read-out.

15 SCISSORS

For cutting away the hair around any wound. These should be curved and round-ended. They must *not* be used for trimming the dog's nails.

16 SPACE BLANKET

To help maintain the dog's body temperature. This is a large sheet of aluminium foil, available at camping and hiking shops. A suitable, though more bulky alternative, is a large sheet of 'bubble wrap'. The blanket must be large enough to cover the dog adequately.

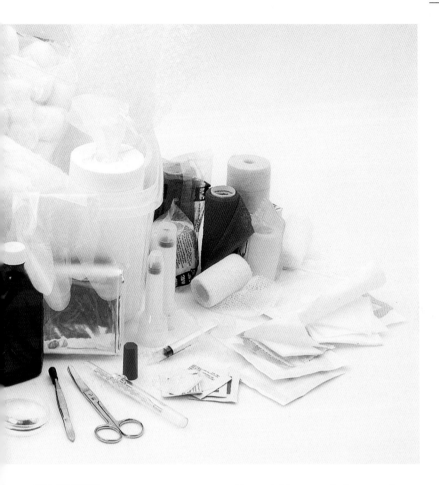

17 STYPTIC PENCIL

To help stem the flow of capillary blood, for example from very minor cuts or bleeding claws and nails. These are available from pharmacists (sold to stem blood flow in humans). Be warned that this will sting the dog, who may react accordingly!

18 SURGICAL GAUZE

For padding wounds and stemming the flow of blood.

19 TABLE SALT   *Saline Solution*

For making into solution. Two teaspoons (approximately 10 ml) of salt mixed in 1 litre (1¾ pints) of warm water is a good solution to wash debris from wounds and counter infection. One teaspoon (approximately 5 ml) of salt mixed in 1 litre (1¾ pints) of warm water with one tablespoon of glucose makes an excellent re-hydrating fluid for dogs. Glucose is a simple sugar, available in powder form from any pharmacy or health food store. The fluid should be given to the dog to drink instead of his normal water. If he will not drink, use a syringe and put the solution directly into the dog's mouth, as you would if you were administering a liquid medicine.

20 TWEEZERS (forceps)

For the removal of foreign bodies. Ensure that these have rounded ends to minimize the chance of injuring the dog. Different lengths may be useful.

Index

a

abdomen distension 27, 116
   Cushing's disease 99
   heart problems 60, 61, 62
   pyometra 82
abscesses 24-5
accidents 102-23
acute moist dermatitis 72
aggression 75
alcohol 69, 120
allergies, food 70
alopecia 65, 67, 77, 99
alveoli 52
anaemia 36, 63, 97
anal adenoma 78
anal foreign bodies 119
anal sac disease 38-9, 91
anorchia 76-7
antihistamine 120
antiseptic lotion 120
appetite
   cravings 96
   increase 28, 29
   insatiable 96
   loss 91, 96
      halitosis 23
      liver failure 94
      mastitis 84
      metritis 86
      pneumonia 57
      renal failure 36
      swallowing difficulties 26-7
arteries 52, 58
arthritis 41, 42, 49, 91, 93
artificial respiration 104, 111, 112, 113
aural discharge 97
aural haematoma 8-9

b

bandages 120
behavioural problems 75-6, 86, 88, 96-7
bitch problems 80-9
bites 117-18

bladder stones 33, 34
bleeding *see* haemorrhage
blindness 21, 91
blood 58-9
breathing 52-7, 107
   anaemia 63
   artificial respiration 104, 111, 112, 113
   heart problems 60, 61, 62
   pneumonia 57
   problems 111-12
bronchioles 52
bronchitis 53, 54, 91
burns 108, 112-13

c

callus pyoderma 72
campylobacter 32, 34
cancer 37, 55, 63, 98
   mammary 83
   testicular 77
   vomiting 30
   see also tumours
capillaries 58
cardiomyopathy 61
cataplexy 114
cataracts 20-1, 28
cervix 80
chemical burns 113
chest compression 104-5, 107, 112
choking 111-12
chronic bronchial disease *see* bronchitis
cilia 52
circulatory system 52, 58-63
coat 64
   hair clipping 117
   problems 91, 92
colitis 32
congenital heart defects 61, 62
conjunctivitis 17, 97
constipation 27, 30, 35, 79, 91
contagious respiratory disease 53
convulsions 113

cornea 16
   ulceration 19
cotton buds 120
cotton wool 120
coughing
   collapsed trachea 56
   heart problems 60, 62
   kennel cough 53
   pneumonia 57
cryptorchidism 76-7
Cushing's disease 73, 99
cyanosis 97
cystitis 33-4, 93, 111

d
deafness 10-11, 91
degenerative disc disease 44-5
dermatitis 72
diabetes insipidus 29
diabetes mellitus 20, 28-9, 30, 34, 73, 97
diarrhoea 30, 32-3, 34-5, 97, 118
   enteritis 34
   liver failure 94
   renal failure 36
digestive system 22-35
dilative cardiomyopathy 61
dislocation 48
drowning 112
dysentery 34

e
ear drum 8, 10
ears
   discharge 97
   flap wounds 14
   foreign bodies 119
   haematoma 8-9
   mites 12, 13, 15
   problems 8-15
   structure 8
eclampsia 85
eczema 72
elderly dogs 90-5
electrocution 113
Elizabethan collar 120
emergencies 102-23
enteritis 33, 34-5
epilepsy 100-1, 113
epiphora 18

euthanasia 101
exercise intolerance 49
   heart problems 62
   pneumonia 57
eyes 16-21
   discharge 97
   foreign bodies 17, 19, 119
   injury 118
   wash 121

f
fainting 118
first aid kit 120-3
fits 113
flatulence 31
fleas 8, 9, 63, 65, 66, 73
folliculitis 65
food allergies 70
foreign bodies 119
   choking 111-12
   conjunctivitis 17
   constipation 35
   corneal ulceration 19
   diarrhoea 32
   epiphora 18
   lameness 41
   otitis 12
   rhinitis 55
   swallowing difficulties 27
   vomiting 30
fractures 46-7, 108, 113-14

g
gastric dilation volvulus complex 116
gastric ulcers 63
gingivitis 23
glaucoma 20
guard hairs 64

h
haemoglobin 59
haemorrhage 63, 97, 105, 110-11, 118
hair 64
   clipping 117
   coat problems 91, 92
   loss see alopecia
halitosis 23, 36, 94
heart
   chest compression 104-5, 107, 112
   disease 27, 91

problems 59-62, 95, 97
structure 59
heart worms 53
heatstroke 30, 111, 113, 114
hip dysplasia 42, 48, 49, 50-1
homeopathy 7
hyperadrenocorticalism 99
hyperplasia 79, 87
hypertrophic cardiomyopathy 61
hypothyroidism 63, 73

i impetigo 72
incontinence 37, 44, 79, 91, 93
inter-digital pyoderma 72
intestines 22
iris 16
iron deficiency 63

j jaundice 97

k kaolin pectate 121
kennel cough 53
kidney failure 30, 34, 36, 63, 91, 97
KY jelly 121

l lameness 40-1, 119
laminectomy 45
leptospirosis 97
lethargy
diabetes 28
pneumonia 57
pyometra 82
lice 63
lifting dogs 108-9
liver failure 27, 30, 63, 91, 94, 97
lymphatic system 58

m male problems 74-9
mammary cancer 83
mange 67
mastitis 84
melting ulcers 19
metritis 86
misalliance 88
mites 8, 12, 13, 15, 67
mitral insufficiency 60, 61
moulting 64

mucus membrane colour 97
muzzle 106, 108, 119, 121-2
myopathy 49
myositis 49

n nails 92
clippers 122
narcolepsy 114
nasal discharge 97
nasal foreign bodies 119
nymphomania 86

o obesity 42, 45, 54, 91, 95
ocular discharge 97
oestrus 80
ossicles 8, 10
osteoarthritis 42, 49, 51
otitis 12-13, 67, 97
otoscope 9, 15
ovaries 80

p pancreas 96
paralysis 43
parvovirus 30, 61
periodontal disease 23, 27
peristalsis 22
phantom pregnancy 28, 80, 81, 97
pharyngitis 26, 27, 39
pharynx 22
pica 96
pinnae 8
plasters 120
pneumonia 57
poisoning 63, 114-16
polydipsia 29, 96-7, 99
polyuria 29, 97, 99
prostate problems 35, 37, 78-9, 93, 111
prostatitis 79
pseudo pregnancy 28, 80, 81, 97
pyoderma 72, 73, 97
pyometra 27, 80, 82, 88

r rat bites 117
renal failure 30, 34, 36
respiratory problems 52-7
retina 16
rhinitis 55

ringworm 70, 71

s salmonella 32
salt 123
scissors 122
seborrhoea 73
senility 91
sexual behaviour 76
    misalliance 88
    nymphomania 86
shock 48, 111, 116
sinusitis 55
skin 64-73
skin-fold pyoderma 72
snake bites 117-18
space blanket 108, 122
spondylosis 42-3
stings 117
stomach 22
styptic pencil 123
surgical gauze 123
swallowing, difficulty 26-7

t tear production 18
teeth 22
    bad breath 23
    broken 24-5, 118
    decay 91, 94
    retained 26
    worn 24-5
temperature 108
tenesmus 32
testes
    anorchia/cryptorchidism 76-7
    tumour 77
thermometer 121, 122
thirst 96-7
    Cushing's disease 99
    diabetes 28, 29
    polydipsia 29, 96-7, 99
    pyometra 82
    renal failure 36
ticks 63, 68-9
tonsillitis 26-7, 39
torsion 30, 116
Toxocara canis 89
trachea 52

    collapsed 56
    traumatic arthritis 42
tumours 19, 99
    anal adenoma 78
    mammary cancer 83
    testes 77
    see also cancer
tweezers 123

u unconsciousness 107, 108
urinary incontinence see incontinence
urolithiasis 34, 37
uterus 80

v vaccinations 53, 97
vagina 80
    discharge 82, 86, 88, 97
    prolapse 87
vaginitis 88, 97
veins 58
vertebral instability 50
vibrissae 64
vitamin deficiency 63
vomiting 27, 30-1, 97, 119
    liver failure 94
    making your dog 115, 116
    mastitis 84
    metritis 86
    pyometra 82
    renal failure 36

w weight loss
    diabetes 28, 29
    heart problems 60, 61, 62
    liver failure 94
    renal failure 36
wet eczema 72
windpipe 52, 56
wobbler's disease 50
wool hairs 64
worms 63, 96, 113
    diarrhoea 32, 33
    heart worms 53
    tapeworms 29
    Toxocara canis 89
    vomiting 30
wounds 14, 108, 110-11, 117, 119

Acknowledgements

Corbis UK Ltd/George Lepp 66.

Sylvia Cordaiy/Anthony Reynolds 48, 67.

John Daniels 23, 39, 68 Top, 68 Bottom, 81 Top, 87, 95, 109 left, 109 right, 110, 121 Top, 121 Centre, 121 Bottom.

Frank Lane Picture Agency/David Dalton 76, /Gerard Laci 74, /Foto Natura 92, /Martin Withers 32, 78.

Octopus Publishing Group Ltd. /Jane Burton 52, 105, 113, 116, 122-123, /Rosie Hyde 21, 33, 36 Bottom, 36-37 Top Centre, 37 right, 57, 65, 72 right /Ray Moller 3, 10, 11, 45 left, /Tim Ridley 6-7, 12.

Angela Hampton/Family Life Picture Library 27, 31, 38 Top Right, 42, 62, 69 Centre, 70, 71, 85 Top, 99, 118.

Jacana/Axel 26, /Susanne Danegger 49, /Durandal 40 Top, /Guy Felix 61, /Michel Garnier 25, /Elizabeth Lemoine 83, /Laurent Borgey Loyer 60, /Mero 28 Top Right, /Michel Viard 51 Top, 56

James McKay 8 Bottom, 9, 13, 14, 16, 22, 40 Bottom, 96, 100, 106 left, 106 Top, 107, 108, 115 Top

RSPCA Photolibrary/Cheryl A Ertelt 15, 41, 45 right, 72 left, /Angela Hampton 19, 29 Bottom Left, 54, 73, 82, 98, 101, /Colin Seddon 94, /John Downer/ Wild Images 75.

Science Photo Library/Eric Grave 29 Top Right, 63, /Robert Holmgren, Peter Arnold Inc. 51 Bottom/Jackie Lewan, EM Unit Royal Free Hospital 89, /Dr Kari Lounatmaa 34, /David Scharf 55

Warren Photographic 81 Centre Right, 90, 117, /Jane Burton 4 Top Right, 4-5, 8 Top, 18, 24, 28 Bottom Left, 30, 38 Bottom Left, 47 Top Left, 47 Centre Left, 47 Bottom, 58, 64, 80, 84, 85 Bottom, 102-103, 104, 111, 115 Centre, /Kim Taylor 69 Bottom.